DATE DUE

FORENSIC ODONTOLOGY

Forensic Odontology

Proceedings of the
European IOFOS Millennium Meeting
Leuven, Belgium
August 23-26, 2000

Edited by

Guy WILLEMS

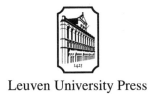

Leuven University Press

I·O·F·O·S

The content of the presentations is not the responsibility of the editor nor of the scientific committee of the European IOFOS Millennium Meeting. The data and opinions appearing in the published material were prepared by and are the responsibility of each of the contributors.

© 2000 by Leuven University Press / Presses Universitaires de Louvain / Universitaire Pers Leuven.
Blijde-Inkomststraat 5, B-3000 Leuven (Belgium)

ISBN 90 5867 051 1
D / 2000 / 1869 / 48

Cover: Lejon Tits

575th ANNIVERSARY K.U.LEUVEN

MISSION STATEMENT JUBILEE

K.U.Leuven, one of the world's oldest catholic universities, celebrates its 575th anniversary in a splendid festive year, which coincides with the dawn of a new millennium. What was visionary and audacious in 1425, has grown into one of today's most comprehensive, famous and international universities of the year 2000. This anniversary is a truly appropriate occasion for K.U.Leuven to demonstrate the grandeur of its past as well as its impact on our present society, but above all to underline its determination to shape tomorrow's world. In the course of many celebrations throughout the year, K.U.Leuven will mark its position in the 21st century as an innovative, inspiring and inquisitive university, actively striving for the fulfilment of humanity's noblest dreams.

The Jubilee will focus on K.U.Leuven's long and rich tradition, as well as on its contribution to the future. This contribution steadily rests on its three pillars. Its leading position in scientific research will be continued and intensified. This research constitutes the basis of its scientific education, the soil of any true university formation. And by its service to society, K.U.Leuven plays an important and versatile role in the development of our society, regionally and nationally as well as internationally. These three pillars are firmly embedded in christian inspiration, ethical re-orientaton and the pursuit of cultural enrichment.

This Jubilee is a period of joyful commemoration and reflection, but more importantly it is also the gateway to the future. K.U.Leuven enters the 21st century as an intellectual, ethical and cultural beacon, pointing to a better world for all.

Preface

As we approach the first year of the new Millennium, many of us get that feeling of becoming part of history. One leg is still in the past but looking ahead, we are hopeful to what the future will bring us. Reflecting over the last century in forensic odontology makes us realise that our roots are visible but small. Amoedo, Gustafson, Ström, Johanson e.a. were the names that many of us grew up with as we took our first steps in the exciting field of forensic odontology. And although evolving quickly, our science is still relatively new, and to some degree under scrutiny.

The Information Super Highway has created exciting opportunities and enables us to obtain information from different fields and different places in virtually no time. Never before has the world seemed so small, and it looks as this is only the beginning of an exciting era of technical innovations, of which we all will benefit to the highest extent. Internet, e-mail, voice mail, teledentistry, speech technology, digital photography and radiology, WAP's have all found or will undoubtedly soon find their way as an application in many fields of our forensic investigations.

But are we as humans developing our minds and spirits at the same Super Highway speed? Are we not letting ourselves be carried away by these evolving techniques rather than listening to our common sense? Are we still critical enough of ourselves and what we do to withstand the pitfalls of this technical revolution? Are we willing to open up our minds and accept the challenges that these evolutions carry with them?

It can not be denied that this Information Super Highway is running in different speeds according to what part of the world we're in. It is the task of those who live in the fast lane to share their knowledge and experience with the less fortunate. Cross breeding has always led to an improvement if the selection of samples is well made, and the techniques are used in a correct way. We must continue to strive to maintain our standards and even raise them to a level equivalent to the new techniques that are being implemented in our investigations.

These are questions, which we will have to face in the near future if we don't want to loose our forensic science credibility.

We cannot deny it though: our background has been one of intuition and anecdote; our future must be one of scientific demonstration and enlightenment.

Eddy De Valck, BDS
IOFOS President
European IOFOS Millennium Meeting President
International Organisation of Forensic Odonto-Stomatology

Contents

List of speakers and chairmen

Benthaus Sven, MD, DDS
Goebenstrasse 73
D-46045 Oberhausen
Germany
swbenthaus@aol.com

Bowers Mike, DDS, JD
2284 S. Victoria Suite 1-G
Ventura
California 93003
USA
cmbowers@aol.com

Braem Marc, DDS, PhD
Universiteit Antwerpen
Department of Dentistry
Groenenborgerlaan 171
B-2020 Antwerpen
Belgium
braem@ruca.ua.ac.be

Cassiman Jean-Jacques, MD, PhD
Katholieke Universiteit Leuven
Faculty of Medicine
Centre for Human Genetics
Herestraat 49
B-3000 Leuven
Belgium

De Valck Eddy, BDS
Parklaan 10
B-1852 Beigem
Belgium
eddy.de.valck@pandora.be

De Winne Joan, Licentiate in
Criminology
Rijkswacht DVI
Ruiterijlaan 2
B-1040 Brussel
Belgium
bs175336@skynet.be

Hill Ian, MD, PhD, LDS
Guy's, King's and St Thomas'
School of Medicine
Guy's Hospital University of
London
Department of Forensic Medicine
SE1 9RT London
Great Britain

Kenney Jack, DDS, MS
101 S. Washington Street
Park Ridge
Illinois 60068-4290
USA
frnscdds@aol.com

Kortelainen Sinikka, DDS, PhD
Health Services
City of Kemi
Kirkkopuistokatu 1
SF-94101 Kemi
Finland
sinikka.kortelainen@kemi.fi

Maat Georges J.R., MD, PhD
Universiteit Leiden
Faculty of Medicine
Wassenaarseweg 72
NL-2333 AL Leiden
The Netherlands
maat@mail.medfac.leidenuniv.nl

Nordblad Anne, DDS, PhD
Stakes
National Research and Development
Centre for Welfare and Health
Siltasaarenkatu 18
P.O. Box 220
SF-00531 Helsinki
Finland
anne.nordblad@stakes.fi

Perrier Michel, DDS, MS
Institut Universitaire de Medecine
Légale
Policlinique Dentaire Universitaire
Rue Dr. Cesar-Roux 23
CH-1005 Lausanne
Switzerland
michel.perrier@chuv.hospvd.ch

Phillips Vince, BDS, MChD
University of Stellenbosch
Private Bag XI
7505 Tygerberg
South Africa
vmp@gerga.sun.ac.za

Prieels Frank, BDS
Bruulstraat 11
B-9450 Haaltert
Belgium
frank.prieels@village.uunet.be

Smeets Bregt, BDS, Licentiate in
Criminology
Dr. Verdurmenstraat 24
B-9100 St. Niklaas
Belgium
bregt.smeets@pandora.be

Solheim Tore, MD, PhD
University of Oslo
Department of Oral Pathology and
Forensic Odontology
P.O. Box 1109 Blindern
N-0317 Oslo
Norway
solheim@odont.uio.no

Sweet David, DMD, PhD
Bureau of Legal Dentistry
146-2355 East Mall
Vancouver, British Columbia
Canada V6T 1Z4
dsweet@unixg.ubc.ca

Taroni Franco, PhD
Institut Universitaire de Médecine
Légale
Université de Lausanne
21, Rue du Bugnon
CH-1005 Lausanne
Switzerland
ftaroni@hola.hospvd.ch

Van de Voorde Wim, MD, PhD
Katholieke Universiteit Leuven
Faculty of Medicine
Centre of Forensic Medicine
Minderbroedersstraat 12
B-3000 Leuven
Belgium
wim.vandevoorde@uz.kuleuven.ac.
be

Vermylen Yvo, BDS, Master in
Laws
Vosweg 23
B-3190 Boortmeerbeek
Belgium
yvovermylen@village.uunet.be

Willems Guy, DDS, PhD
Katholieke Universiteit Leuven
Faculty of Medicine
School of Dentistry, Oral Pathology
and Maxillofacial Surgery
Department of Orthodontics
Kapucijnenvoer 7
B-3000 Leuven
Belgium
guy.willems@uz.kuleuven.ac.be

Wood R.E., DDS, MSc, PhD
University Health Network
Princess Margaret Hospital
Department of Dental Oncology
Dental and Maxillofacial Radiology
610 University Avenue
Toronto, Ontario
Canada M5G 2M9
rwood@cgo.wave.ca

Bang Gisle, MD, PhD
Haukeland hospital
Department of Oral Pathology and
Forensic Odontology
N-5021 Bergen
Norway

21ˢᵗ century quality standards in forensics

Quality standards related to forensics in general dentistry

A. Nordblad

STAKES - FINLAND
NATIONAL RESEARCH AND DEVELOPMENT CENTRE FOR WELFARE AND HEALTH
SERVICES AND QUALITY

Drafting and keeping patient documents

In Finland the provisions of the Act (785/92) concerning the position and rights of patients apply in relation to the duty of health care professionals to prepare and maintain patient documents, and keep the information in them confidental. Provisions concerning confidentiality notwithstanding, each health care professional must provide declarations, explanations and clarifications requested by the National Board of Medico-Legal Affairs or a provincial administrative board necessary for performance of the duties prescribed under this Act. Each health care professional must take out insurance as prescribed in the Patient Injury Act (585/86).

Health care professionals and each health care unit shall draft and keep patient documents in the way prescribed more precisely by the Ministry of Social Affairs and Health. According to the Act concerning health care professionals

(559/94) the professional activities of health care professionals should be directed towards the promotion and maintenance of health, the prevention of illness, and the curing of those who are ill, and alleviation of their suffering. In his or her professional activities, a health care professional must employ generally accepted, empirically justified methods, in accordance with his or her training which must be continually supplemented. In his or her professional activity, each health care professional must weigh benefits and hazards to the patient. Health care professionals must take account of stipulations concerning patients' rights.

Finnish national set of quality recommendations in Social Welfare and Health Care

The second national set of recommendations - Quality Management in Social Welfare and Health Care for the 21st Century - attempts to meet the challenges to quality management in the Finnish social welfare and health care sector. The recommendations apply to both public and private social welfare and health care services. In addition to service providers, important contributors include customer and professional organisations, bodies responsible for quality management within training and persons conducting research on quality management.

The recommendations encourage the involvement of customers in quality management. More attention is paid to the role of preventive activities in the promotion of well being and health than what was the case in the previous set of recommendations. Emphasis is placed on the management of internal and external processes and on a systematic way of doing things - aspects that can be improved by means of many different techniques. The importance of information in the assessment of quality and the achievement of higher quality continues to be stressed. Emphasis is also placed on quality criteria as tools in quality management and monitoring.

A customer-centred approach is today a more widely accepted objective in the development of public and private services than was formerly the case, and it is one of the basic ideas of administrative reform. Close co-operation between customer and professional results in genuine mutual influence and dialogue between equal partners. Patient and customer organisations also have an important role in pointing out the needs of special groups.

Ever more frequently, quality must be demonstrated by means of well-conducted internal or external assessments. The staff of organisations in the social welfare and health care sector must be adequate in number and appropriately trained. In some fields, formal qualification requirements have been defined quite strictly at the legislative level. They do not, however, guarantee sufficient competence: staff members need adequate opportunities for guidance in their work and for further training aimed at updating the knowledge and skills acquired during their basic training. As well as professional expertise, such training should cover skills required for quality management, since these are not yet comprehensive within the basic training. Supplementary training aimed at maintaining and increasing professional competence should be based on an evaluation of what is needed for the development of activities, teams and processes.

As far as the basic professional content is concerned, service lines and chains are steered by good operating practices, by recommendations for action and care and by regional care programs. These can be used as a basis for the evaluation of processes. The quickest way to change activities so that they conform to evidence-based recommendations for action and care is to change processes.

Correct handling of personal data

Important components in relations with the customer/patient and of service quality are the correct handling of personal data and adherence to regulations concerning the maintaining of personal records. The right of service users to enjoy privacy and to determine what may be done with data concerning them highlights the importance of recorded information and of users' consent with regard to the way in which personal data is handled. The information contained in the records of service providers and regional and national bodies must contain no errors and must provide objective information on a particular case. The body maintaining the records is responsible for the appropriateness of entries. Service users may have entries amended by making use of their right to inspect records and to demand that errors be rectified. The leadership of service providers is responsible for training staff in the correct handling of personal data.

Operating systems to suit organisations

In the case of small organisations or one-person providers, quality can be managed using simpler procedures and guiding principles than those needed in larger organisations. A large, multilevel organisation needs correspondingly more operation guidelines, process descriptions and quality management methods if it is to achieve the desired results.

A general characteristic of a good quality system is that processes have been documented and have been specified so as to meet minimum demands as far as the satisfaction of customers' needs is concerned. Staff has been trained so that they understand the purpose of the described procedures. In addition, steps have been taken to ensure that the system functions well and can be developed. An organisation can assess its own quality management and the effectiveness of its quality system. Such cases are described as self-assessments or internal assessments (or often audits). In the case of self-assessments, one can use self-defined criteria or some existing set of criteria - for example, the self-assessment method (ITE) developed by the Association of Finnish Local and Regional Authorities, the criteria of the King's Fund method, sets of criteria for quality awards or the ISO 9000 criterion sets.

Use of the dental record in quality assessment

Although appropiate records do not ensure the adequacy of dental care, they provide an opportunity to evaluate it, while poor records do not (Jerge and Orlowski, 1985). The patient record is a legal document and is the basis for judgement in matters of responsibility and malpractice. Yet the quality of dental patient records is not always acceptable (Forsberg, 1992; Rasmusson et al., 1994). In forensic odontology information in the patient document constitutes the ante mortem information which is compared to post mortem information about the deceased during identification. An incomplete patient record may hamper forensic odontology casework and the success in identification stands or falls with the existence of comparable ante mortem and post mortem data (Keiser-Nielsen, 1977). According to quality evaluation of patient records in Swedish dental care, Swedish dental patient records constitute poor ante mortem material for forensic odontology (Rasmusson et al., 1994). The conclusion was that the standard of the patient record must be improved.

National Research and Development Centre for Welfare and Health (Stakes) together with seven Health Care Centres in different parts of Finland started a project of quality management of dental health care services for handicapped patients in 1995. An important part of the project was to evaluate the quality of the patient records by auditing and then implement necessary improvements. The quality of patient records in oral health care has not been previously studied in Finland.

Material and methods

As a part of quality project, a first round to audit patient records was done during the spring 1996 in seven health care centres. A total of 423 patient records were evaluated in the first audit round. The local dental team in each of the seven health care centres did the audit. The analyses of the results were done at the University of Kuopio. The results were analysed by different health care centres and feedback was given to each health care centre separately. Health care centres did arrange training of the personnel and the results were studied in each health centre and procedures for improvement were determined.

The second audit was done during the year 1998. On total 383 patient records were evaluated again by second audit. The same standardised form was used as in the first audit in 1996. The questionnaire consisted of 37 questions of patients, therapy measures, diagnosis, prognosis etc..

Results

The frequency of correct documentation for some selected parameters is shown in Table 1. The identity of the patient was completed in the second audit in all the records with exception of two records. Certain rules, such as documentation of a name of the professional, patient identity, dental health status and detailed record notes of the given care corresponding patient's need were followed by most dentists. Documentation of therapy plans, anamnestic findings and summaries of the treatment/care were reported more rarely.

Table 1: Results of the frequencies of correct documentation of parameters in accordance with Finnish regulations of patient records in first auditing in 1996 compared with the second auditing in 1998 (n = number of investigated patient records)

Parameter	1996	n	1998	n
Care giver identity noted	100 %	429	100 %	367
Professional identity noted	77 %	429	86 %	367
Patient identity noted	95 %	429	99 %	367
Custodian noted	74 %	429	87 %	367
Documentation of anamnestic findings	46 %	429	73 %	366
Documentation of status	94 %	429	99 %	366
Radiographs have been taken	36 %	429	31 %	364
Documentation of diagnoses	68 %	429	82 %	365
Documentation of therapy plan	48 %	429	82 %	365
Summary of the treatment	18 %	424	46 %	363
Detailed record notes on care	91 %	194	95 %	364

Conclusions

The present study carried in Finland showed that even though the quality of patient records in dental clinics are often inadequate, a great improvement can be achieved with quality management and auditing process. Our results showed that the information in the patient records was not in accordance with the rules for the patient records given by the Ministry of Social Affairs and Health. After audits and training of the personnel better recordings were achieved in our project. However, the need remains for improvement of patient recording accuracy in dentistry in Finland. In order to improve quality management in the social welfare and health care sector and to provide support for persons and organisations involved in such work, a start has been made in 1999 with the publication of quality management support materials such as a handbook of a good practise of drafting patient documents in oral health care.

References

Forsberg H. (1992) Hur förs journaler inom vuxentandvården? En pilotstudie utförd på tre tandvårdskliniker i Norrbotten. Klinikbaserad kvalitetssäkring inom tandvården. Rapport från konferens socialstyrelsen.

Jerge C.R. and Orlowski R.M. (1985) Quality assurance and the dental record. *Dental Clinics of North America* **29**: 483-96.

Keiser-Nielsen S. (1977) Person identification by means of the teeth. A practical guide. John Wright & Sons Ltd., Bristol, United Kingdom.

National Recommendation. (1999) Quality Management in Social Welfare and Health Care for the 21st Century. Ministry of Social Affairs and Health, National Research and Development Centre for Welfare and Health (Stakes) and Association of Finnish Local and Regional Authorities.

Rasmusson L., René N., Dahlbom U., Borrman H. (1994) Quality evaluation of patient records in Swedish dental care. *Swedish Dental Journal* **18**: 233-41.

What does the law say?

E. De Valck

DISASTER VICTIM IDENTIFICATION TEAM - BELGIUM
CHIEF FORENSIC ODONTOLOGIST

Introduction

The availability and accuracy of the dental records is very often a crucial factor in the identification of unknown individuals and corpses. In some of the investigations that forensic odontologists participate in as dental experts they have to establish an identity of one or more unknown persons or corpses. In such cases they often have to deal with the ante mortem dental record of the deceased or missing persons in order to make a comparison for identification. Very frequently one of the main problems is to obtain these ante mortem records, for a variety of reasons. One might be because the investigators cannot establish the identity of the victim's practitioner. Sometimes they get as far as the dentist but cannot get their hands on the dental records because they either have been destroyed, or are not stored, or are just not being kept by the dentist. And even if the dental records are obtained we might still find ourselves faced with incomplete or insufficient ante mortem dental records jeopardising the results of our investigations.

In order to obtain usable dental records in forensic investigations it might be necessary that governments create a legal framework in which the dentist will be required to keep dental records. If the government is failing to fulfil its duties to society, it should be the Dental Board's duty to create a code of ethics, which would not have the force of legislation, but would clearly be a good guide to the ethics of the dental profession.

Legal and ethical considerations

Dental practitioners in every European country have to respect legal and ethical principles. Whether formally expressed as laws, oaths or as written guidelines these principles relate to their relationship with patients, other dentists and the wider public.

The most common method of providing dentists with ethical guidance is through a simple written code. This is usually administered by the national dental association, or in some countries by a separate regulating body (e.g. in Ireland, U.K., France). The application of these codes is usually by committees at a local level. Dentists' professional and other behaviours are usually also governed by specific laws (Dental Acts e.g. in Norway, Iceland), more general medical laws (e.g. Italy; Austria where dentists must take the 'Hippocratic Oath') as well as laws on professional and business conduct.

As a lot of jurisprudence of dental records keeping runs parallel for dental and medical records, we believe that we can agree upon the statement made in an early Western Australian case: 'Prudent practice demands that a proper record of the treatment should be noted immediately' (Henson v Perth Hosp Management Bd, 1939). In a similar fashion this was also stated by a Canadian court in Kolesar v Jeffries. 'Medical records are an important tool in the practice of medicine. They serve as a base for planning patient care; they provide a means of communication between the attending physician and other physicians and with nurses and other professional groups contributing to the patient's care; they furnish documentary evidence of the course of the patient's illness, treatment and response to treatment... (and) they serve as the basic document for the medical staff's review, study and evaluation of the medical care rendered to the patient'.

Whatever jurisdiction one looks at, the picture is always the same: courts dislike poorly kept records. Badly kept records create a generally poor impression of the provided care, while well-kept records may in themselves provide an index (though not a warranty) of good dental care and, as a matter of defendant's credibility, may protect him from civil liability.

In 1994 the Dental Board of South Australia, because of the seriousness of the particulars alleged, terminated three inquiries into unprofessional conduct and laid complaints itself to the Professional Dental Conduct Tribunal. It became evident from observing these proceedings how critical the keeping of accurate and contemporary dental records was to the Tribunal's judgement.

It is abundantly clear from available case law that records should be kept on all patients (Cagnon v Stortini, 1974, where a dentist kept records only of his 'regular patients', and not of those who came in on a 'casual or emergency' basis), and that they must be accurate, objective and contemporary with the event recorded as possible, and complete.

In some jurisdictions, these requirements are set out by statute and in others by the courts, but the message is the same: The records must give all necessary information about the patient's identity; contain all the necessary medical history and diagnosis information, contain all the information about received treatment.

Although it is not common standard yet, a number of countries do have legal regulations on this matter. Since Sweden, in addition to legislation, has instructions for dental records issued by the Swedish National Board of Health and Welfare (SOFS), Borrman et al. (1995) studied the quality of dental records used for identification purposes between 1983 and 1992. The most revealing result of the investigation was that 94% of the records were incomplete on previous therapy. Also in only 40 % of the records the available radiographs in the dental record could be identified.

A personal questionnaire was sent out inquiring about the existence of laws or regulations keeping dental records. Out of 60 countries, 28 responded. In 18 countries there were regulations on keeping dental records, but only in 13 was stipulated what the content of the dental record had to be. The time that these records had to be kept varied between 2 – 30 years and only 1 country provides extra remuneration for the work done.

In Belgium, the situation is handled by the Ministry of Health and the Ministry of Social Affairs. Recently a proposal has been made, where patients over 60 years benefit financially from a system in which their full medical record is managed and kept by a health care provider of their choice. Up to the end of 1999 about 450.000 patients had decided to join the system. The record keeper receives a small financial compensation on an annual basis.

Attempts have been made by dentists active in forensics to introduce a law or regulation on dental records, but it seems to take a long way to convince the decision makers at different levels of the dental association and government of the necessity of such requirement.

Contents of the records

Exemplary record keeping is as important to the health care system itself as it is to the patient and the practitioner. The dentist's primary ethical and legal responsibility is to offer a service which is in the patient's best interest, and proper record keeping is part of that obligation. And even though much is said of the duty of care owed by a dentist to his or her patients, dentists also have a primary duty of care to themselves, to keep appropriate records.

All records should be dated, accurate and legible, and made at the time the examination or treatment is carried out.

In our recent survey mentioned above on regulations regarding the content of dental records 13 countries described the situation in detail. A lot of what is required runs parallel and serves the same purpose.

Minimum requirements of the content are:
- the patient's full name, address, date of birth;
- the dentist's identification;
- dental and medical history to be updated at every visit;
- existing status of the dentition at the first visit;
- clinical records (medication, treatment, anaesthetics, materials);
- radiographs (to be labelled with patient's name, date);
- signature of the dentist at each note;
- unusual characteristics;
- referrals to colleagues and the answers;
- correspondence about the patient.

Within this patient-dentist relationship, the dentist requires data from the patient in order to provide proper advice and treatment, and the patient has the responsibility to co-operate by providing such data properly, correctly and as fully as necessary. The patient will assume that this confidential communication with the practitioner will not be revealed to third parties.

Confidentiality of the record

The duty of non-disclosure of confidential information is laid down in the 'Hippocratic Oath' and, in a modern version in the Declaration of Geneva (1947), as amended in Sydney in 1968 and Venice in 1983, as well as in various national professional rules, regulations and statutes providing for the confidentiality of data derived within a the patient-practitioner relationship.

Indeed, a practitioner who violates this duty of secrecy by making (but unauthorised) disclosures may be indicted for a criminal offence – most Penal Codes provide sentences – or subjected to disciplinary proceedings by his professional board.

This duty is of an on-going nature and it does not cease with the conclusion of the dentist-patient relationship or the death of the patient or doctor.

Some concerns have been expressed recently about the authorised transfer of patient data in our 21st century information technology society. The problem of protected transfer of patient data through the intranet/internet has to be seriously considered if the confidentiality of the data has to be respected.

Telemedicine/teledentistry may lead to civil and professional law suits if confidentiality securing protective systems are not built in.

Some breaches of confidence are, however, authorised by statue. For example, dental records can be summoned for court proceedings and coronal investigations.

When the dentist is acting as an expert, he is only allowed to reveal that part of the content of the records which is directly related to the task he has been assigned within the expert's requisitory.

Access to and ownership of the record

As a general rule, no record may be revealed or made accessible to anyone without the patient's consent. This general rule follows from the very personal nature of the data obtained, which is also protected by the practitioner's duty and right, to maintain confidentiality. This means that the records have to be protected at all time for third parties, and can only be revealed upon legal request.

The legal position is that records are, and remain, the property of the dental practitioner who compiled them at the institution in which the patient was treated. The practitioner is under no obligation to provide these records to the patient, who is legally the 'owner' of the content of the records. If requested a copy of the original record should be provided to the patient. Not all information on the record should necessarily be revealed to the patient, but only that part which is in relation to the patient's treatment. Personal information available on the record can be withheld.

The record must also be made available to succeeding practitioners treating the patient upon the patient's request. The practitioner may be held liable for failing to provide records to a patient's succeeding practitioner.

When a dental practitioner dies or retires, his or her practice may continue under the supervision of new or existing dentists who are part of that practice. The records remain generally within the practice. If he or she dies they become the property and responsibility of the executor of the estate. They must be retained, and of course the duty of confidentiality remains.

How long should records be retained?

The legislation on this matter varies from one country to another as was observed in our recent inquiry. The time varies between 2 and 30 years, with a range between 5 and 10 years as the most common. For children's records it is often necessary to keep them for this period of time after the child has become an adult.

Often these periods have been determined on an arbitrary base to bear some relation to the possibility of litigation. This arbitrary rule of thumb may not necessarily be appropriate, particularly when one considers the forensic importance of dental records.

Burton 'Medical Ethics and Law' (Giesen, 1988) suggests that ' the real test seems to be whether destruction of medical and dental records by a practitioner might constitute a breach of duty of core owed to his patient. Even when the dentist/patient relationship has ceased ant the patient is under the care of another practitioner, the records may be important for future reference for the purpose of dental care or to establish legal rights.

This length of time to retain dental records is extremely important in the cases of missing persons. When an individual is reported missing the police officer at the CBO (Centraal Bureau Opsporingen – Missing and unidentified persons Service) will register statements relating to the person's personal characteristics. In jurisdictions where it is legal to do so, also the missing person's medical and dental records will be collected and added to the profile.

If the individual has been missing for a long time and has not seen a dentist in the period prior to its disappearance, the chances will be good that the dental record is no longer available at the practitioner's office since there is no law or regulation that forces the dentist to keep these records.

Conclusions

The availability of complete, accurate and comprehensive treatment dental records is an ethical, and in some countries a legal obligation of the dentist. It is not only a duty to the patient and the base for appropriate treatment, but at the same time a primary duty of care to themselves to protect them against litigation.

Although some countries do have laws and ethical regulations these rules are not always followed by dentists. This could lead to liability suit from the patient but also to professional law suits from dental authorities.

One could even raise the question when the day will come that a dentist who fails to keep appropriate dental records despite a legal obligation will be suited by the family of a non identifiable person because of the lack of this kind of information.

References

Bell G.L. (1997) Missing and Unidentified Persons: A disaster of immense Magnitude. *American Society of Forensic Odontology News* Summer, pp. 20-22.

Borrman H., Dahlbom U, Loyola E., René N. (1995) Quality evaluation of 10 years patient records in forensic odontology. *International Journal of Legal Medicine* **108**: 100-104.

Dorion R. (1997) FBI Task Force to enhance Dental Coding Standards. *American Society of Forensic Odontology News* Winter, pp.4-5.

EU Manual of Dental Practice (1997) © Member Associations of the Dental Liaison Committee in the EU.

Giesen D. (1988) International Medical Malpractice Law. Martinus Nijhoff Publishers, Dordrecht, The Netherlands

Quality assurance guidelines for post mortem identification

S. Benthaus*, K. Rötzscher*, B. Knell**, H. Van Waes**, J. Bonnetain***, J. Hutt***

* Disaster Victim Identification team - Germany
** Association of Forensic Dentists - Switzerland
*** Association Française d'Identification Odontologique - France

Introduction

The identification of unknown individuals plays a social and forensic role (Endris, 1982). Not only is it of importance to the relatives, it also provides the basis for criminological investigations and for those relating to insurance law and penal law.

The major significance of positive identification makes exact, objectively lucid and scientifically founded investigative methods essential. Only adherence to generally binding quality assurance guidelines can lead in individual cases and in mass disasters to identification expertises capable of withstanding legal and judicial scrutiny and offering an indispensable degree of scientific reliability.

It must also be borne in mind that achievements in the transportation sector coupled with the ever-increasing mobility of the individual resulted in a growing number of large-scale disasters. They represent a substantial destruction potential to society and make an internationally binding standard for post mortem identification after mass disasters mandatory.

For instance, the number of fatalities in aircraft accidents in 1996 was 1840, with the number of passengers having undergone a 75% increase between 1976 and 1996. Air travel thus produces disasters of a new type, disasters which are not only characterised by the high degree of individual fragmentation or destruction but whose scene is set increasingly on international terrain.

Fourteen out of 20 deployments by the Identification Commission of the Federal German Bureau of Criminal Investigation (Interpol - Germany) have taken place outside Germany. Mass disasters on an international scale, such as the 1997 Luxor shootings involving victims from seven different countries, make international on-the-spot co-operation among investigating authorities and forensic experts essential. This stresses the need for an international standard when dealing with mass disasters.

Besides a uniform international nomenclature, a standardised system of recording and documenting post mortem findings represents an indispensable precondition for successful identification, especially in cases involving foreign nations.

Recording of findings

With the investigating authorities endeavouring to complete post mortem identification in the shortest possible time, the investigator is in search of features which offer a high degree of individual specificity and post mortem stability and which are documented for broad sections of the population during their lifetime (Benthaus, 1977). Well protected in the oral cavity from the influence of external force, the jaws and teeth meet these requirements exceptionally well. Together with morphological differences, pathological and restorative changes to the dental system often represent adequate identity markers. A complete dentition provides 3.8×10^4 restoration states (Hausmann et al., 1977). Despite the increased incidence of certain findings in the dentition, the degree of individual specificity can be assumed to be adequate (Friedmann et al., 1989), and even naturally healthy dentitions with no fillings reveal morphological structures with a high degree of individual specificity.

At each stage of post mortem identification, it must be borne in mind that any supplementary procedure (biochemical analysis, materials analysis, facial reconstruction etc.) may be rendered not only more difficult but even impossible by inappropriate action.

Embedded in the orofacial soft tissue, the teeth and jaws are not accessible for simple visual post mortem inspection. Whenever the complete post mortem dental findings are to be recorded, it is therefore advisable to perform a full resection of both jaws (Heidemann, 1988), as this is the only means of recording complete findings. Exceptionally small identity markers and enamel-matched fillings may be overlooked during intraoral inspection due to contamination by blood and putrescence. Incorrect and incomplete findings may lead to serious cases of misidentification (Brown, 1982). For this reason it is now considered inadequate to leave the jaw in situ. In our opinion, the right of the deceased person to an unequivocal identity determined with absolute certainty outweighs any moral misgivings against excision of the jaws. In all events, the decision on removal is in the hands of the competent public prosecutor, who has to be informed of the significance of this recommended procedure.

Autopsy techniques have been described in literature (Endris, 1979; Fereira et al., 1997; Rötzscher, 1998). Following transbuccal access, the maxilla is chiselled or sawn out in the Le Fort I plane, with care being taken to protect the tooth roots. It is vital to prevent any damage to the root apices. Only in exceptional cases should the mandible be completely disarticulated, and osteotomised distal of the dentition in the angle of the mandible, in order not to aggravate the situation in the event of the mandible being needed for facial soft tissue reconstruction.

If more than one body is being examined simultaneously, it is essential to use clear-cut markings and separate storage facilities to exclude any risk of mistaken identity. As advanced putrescence may result in severe loosening of monoradicular teeth in particular, special care must be taken in the subsequent cleaning process to ensure that no further teeth are lost post mortem. Deep-freezing autopsy specimens allows re-examination at any time without the body having to be exhumed. Maceration of the jaws provides long-life specimens characterised by high quality and constant availability. Prior to maceration, however, DNA samples and material for biochemical analysis (age determination) should be collected, since chemical maceration may rule out the use of these techniques.

For the recording of findings, the artefacts should be placed on the autopsy table in such a way as to provide a frontal view into the oral cavity. This procedure eliminates the risk of the two sides being inadvertently confused. In addition to the number of teeth and the location of fillings and of prosthetic appliances, data have to be recorded on the general state of the dentition, abrasion facets and filling materials used.

Once the native preparations have been photographed, enamel-matched restorations can be located with the enamel-staining method, a technique that reliably eliminates any risk of confusion between filling margins and fissures in the enamel.

Radiographic technique

The radiograph reveals not only fillings and pathological changes in the dental system but also morphological characteristics of the bones and teeth. Conformity between ante mortem and post mortem radiographs may therefore pave the way to positive identification. The benefit of radiographic comparison has been underlined in numerous judicial enquiries. If dental radiographs are available at the time of abduction, efforts should be made to reproduce the ante mortem projection parameters as far as possible for post mortem radiography to permit a „like with like" comparison (Whittaker and McDonald, 1993). The position of the film in relation to the tooth is determined in part by anatomical structures: the floor of the mouth, the tongue, the lips and the palatal vault. The facial and oral soft tissue components thus make an inevitable contribution to both ante mortem and post mortem film positioning, so that the surrounding soft tissue can be utilised as one factor in film positioning. The jaws can be x-rayed before or after removal. Good results can be achieved with either method, subject to adequate experience. If the soft tissue is intact, exposure times should be adapted to those for living patients. However, if the soft tissue covering is lost, the exposure time is reduced by 25 % to 50 %, using the same tube voltage. Our own investigations have shown that radiography alone is inadequate for the localisation of enamel-matched filling materials.

A forensic odontological examination not including post mortem radiography of the teeth and jaws has to be regarded as inadequate and thus as defective in individual cases. Cecchi et al. reported in 1997 on the incorrect identification of a military pilot who had been shot down in 1986 during a deployment in northern Africa. A few months later, a body in an advanced state of putrefaction was found. The fact that the pilot and his copilot had a clinically identical dental status had led to the initial misidentification. It was only three years later that radiographic comparison revealed that the body was not that of the pilot but that of his copilot.

Photographic recording of findings

The post mortem findings are secured by photographing the artefacts in frontal and oblique lateral view in occlusal position from both sides prior to removal of the jaws. These photos are then supplemented by topographical occlusal projections. The guiding principle is always that, as a precautionary measure, several photos of each view are taken with varying imaging parameters to allow for incorrect exposure or reflected glare. For further reference it is important to include in the photo a right-angled scale plus a clear-cut investigation number. For this purpose the American Board of Forensic

Odontology has developed a scale made of non-reflecting plastic, which minimises photographic distortion.

State-of-the-art reflex cameras with TTL metering systems and ring flash systems (Benthaus, 1998), as are used in clinical photography, lend themselves to forensic applications. For mass disaster management purposes, Polaroid photos are recommended for their immediate availability.

Written recording of findings - Interpol form and anatomical dental record

As early as 1988, Interpol responded to the growing number of mass diasters by setting up an international commission for the identification of disaster victims. The factors underlying successful data exchange on an international scale are a fixed nomenclature and the use of internationally standardised forms such as the INTERPOL form, which has been used successfully in Norway for a number of years, even for individual cases. The form can be filled in by means of a Windows program and fed into a comparative database or into the Internet.

The Interpol form should be supplemented in all events by an anatomical dental record. The Swiss ID Form is ideal for this purpose. Hemisectioned teeth, post abutments, root fillings and morphological root characteristics cannot be correctly recorded except in an anatomical dental record.

Two dental experts working independently of each other should record the findings, and the result should be documented in an examination report signed by both experts.

NMR (Numerical-Morphological-Radiographic) Certainty Index

Dental identification should be carried out by qualified forensic odontologists only. Analysis of comparative data is the most difficult part of odontological identification and the result of the examination must be unequivocal in its formulation and must provide a clear-cut statement on the identity of the person concerned. As early as 1977, Keiser-Nielsen (1977a) emphasised the need to evaluate the comparative data recorded according to the frequency of features. Andersen et al. (1995) classified the ante mortem data into five categories. Experience has shown that single features have a sufficient degree of individual specificity: this applies in particular to radiographic comparison. We therefore propose that a numerical, morphological and radiographic quality code should be specified in the expertise for quality assurance purposes.

This would prevent individual identity markers with an unknown frequency from being overrated in a population. A description of the minimum requirements is deliberately renounced, as individual identity markers, too, may have a sufficiently high degree of individual specificity to meet identification requirements without additional factors.

The NMR Index (Table 1) comprises all scientifically verifiable comparative parameters on which the identity statement is based. This enables the expert to evaluate the reliability of his findings and to carry out supplementary investigations if necessary.

Table 1: N(umerical) M(orphological) R(adiographic) Certainty Index

Parameter	Description
N_0	No numerical conformity, but no contradiction
N_1	Numerical conformity
M_0	No morphological conformity, but no contradiction
M_{1-x}	Number of unequivocally morphological conforming structures (filling etc.)
R_0	No radiographic comparison possible
R_{1-x}	Number of radiographically conforming structures

Example 1

Post mortem examination reveals the absence of teeth 12 and 35. The comparative material provided by the Bureau of Criminal Investigation comprises a dental status dating back several years, in which tooth 35 is likewise missing. There are no entries concerning fillings, and no radiographs.

Comparison of the ante mortem and post mortem data would undoubtedly be insufficient per se for unequivocal identification. The findings correspond to group N_0, M_0, R_0: no numerical conformity, but no contradiction, no morphological or radiographic conformity. Additional investigations would be absolutely indispensable.

Example 2

In another case, the post mortem findings likewise reveal the absence of teeth 12 and 35. Tooth 35 is missing in the ante mortem dental status too. Post mortem examination reveals two mesio-occluso-distal fillings, and a root filling in tooth 46 can be identified by comparing the ante mortem and post mortem radiographs.

The lack of numerical conformity (two missing teeth post mortem; one missing tooth ante mortem) can be accounted for without contradiction by an extraction performed at a later date (N_0). Two fillings conform in location and scope (M_2). Radiographic comparison of the root filling in tooth 46 reveals a high degree of individual specificity (R_1). Identification can be regarded as certain. Verifiable scientific criteria can be documented as $N_0M_2R_1$ certainty. No further examinations are required.

According to recommendations by Keiser-Nielsen (1977b), 12 morphological conformities are necessary for identification with absolute certainty, whereas one single radiographic comparison is sufficient for this purpose. Numerical conformities alone are not sufficient for identification.

Verifiability, authenticity, storage of artefacts, filing of odontological identification documents

The great significance of the identity of a person beyond his death was outlined in the introduction. In view of this significance, it is clear that all materials relating to the identification of an unknown individual (artefacts, DNA material and comparative material, ante mortem and post mortem findings, radiographs, expertises) must be stored with the greatest care. Special attention must be paid to the authenticity of the comparative material provided. The decision on the duration of the record keeping has to be taken by the investigating authorities in consultation with the competent public prosecutor.

References

Benthaus S. (1977) Systematik der Röntgenidentifikation. *Archives für Kriminologie* **200**: 95-106.

Benthaus S. (1998) Ringblitz-Seitenblitz Kombination - eine sinnvolle Ergänzung für die zahnärztliche Fotographie? *Quintessenz* **49**: 69-72.

Brown K. (1982) The identification of Linda Agostini. *American Journal of Forensic Medicine and Pathology* **3**: 131-141.

Cecchi R., Cipolloni L., Nobile M. (1997) Incorrect identification of a military pilot with international implications. *International Journal of Legal Medicine* **110**: 167-169.

Endris R. (1979) Praktische Forensische Odontostomatologie. Kriminalistik Verlag, Heidelberg.

Endris R. (1982) Forensische Katastrophenmedizin. Identifizierungskommissionen. Kriminalistik Verlag, Heidelberg.

Fereira J., Ortega A., Avila A., Espina A., Leendertz R., Barrios F. (1997) Oral autopsy of unidentified burned human remains. *American Journal of Forensic Medicine and Pathology* **18**: 306-311.

Friedmann R.B., Cornwell K.A., Lorton L. (1989) Dental characteristics of a large military population useful for identification. *Journal of Forensic Sciences* **34**: 1357-1364.

Hausmann R., Liebler M., Schellmann B. (1997) Zur Personenidentifikation mittels Zahnstatus. *Rechtsmedizin* **7**: 86-89.

Heidemann D. (1988) Identifizierungsarbeiten in Ramstein. *Zahnärztliche Mitteilungen* **78**: 2116-2123.

Keiser-Nielsen S. (1977a) Dental Identification: Certainty v. Probability. *Forensic Science International* **9**: 87-97.

Keiser-Nielsen S. (1977b) Person identification by means of the teeth. A practical guide. John Wright & Sons Ltd., Bristol, United Kingdom.

Rötzscher K. and Solheim (1998) Organization der Identifizierung. In: Identifikation unbekannter Toter. Leopold D., ed. Verlag Schmidt Römhild, Lübeck.

Whittaker D. and McDonald G. (1993) Atlas der Forensischen Zahnmedizin. Dr. Ärzte Verlag, Cologne, Germany.

The liability of the forensic odontologist

Y. Vermylen

The expert-witness

An 'expert' can be defined as one who has acquired special knowledge of the subject matter about which he has to testify, either by study, education or practical experience, and who can assist and guide the jury and the judge in solving a problem which would otherwise remain unsolved because of the inadequate knowledge of jury and judge.

A witness, who by education and/or experience has become an expert in any art, science, profession or calling may be permitted to state his opinion as to the matter in which he is versed and which is material to the case, and he may also state his reasons.

Experts have a privileged position among witnesses in the court system, both in the civil law and common law tradition. They are allowed to give expert evidence in the form of opinion in much broader circumstances than lay witnesses on the meaning and implications of other evidence.

Selection or appointment of expert-witness

In civil law countries a court magistrate, a judge of instruction or a trial judge of the criminal court appoints experts. If the judge decides that you are an expert, then you are an expert. Experts are chosen from official or semi-official lists. To become an expert, one can apply for recognition by the court. The only investigation performed by the courts is make sure that you don't have a criminal record and that you are fit for the job. If you have a dental diploma, you may apply for the job of forensic odontologist. The courts do not investigate your education, practical experience in the field or personal training.

The above mentioned legal authorities decide what the exact content of your mission as an expert will be. They have the power to give the expert specific instructions about the task he has to fulfil in order to advise them about the facts of the crime.

The investigation of the crime and also the work done by the expert is written and secret until the case is ready to be handled by the court. The expert makes his report and that report is filed in the record of the case. The expert can be convoked to testify in court, to demonstrate or to clarify his report.

There is no examination-in-chief, no cross-examination or re-examination. His qualifications are never contested and reports of an expert for the defense are rather a curiosity than a rule.

In common law countries experts are selected by the prosecution or the defense. The expert can become involved in different phases of the dispute:
-    His most important contribution is situated in the pre-trial phase when it has to be decided if there is a case and whether it is better to seek an out-of-court settlement or to proceed with litigation after an investigation of the strength or weakness of the evidence of the case.
-    Give technical assistance to the legal team
-    Advise on the meaning and significance of opposing evidence
-    Give evidence at the hearing

The procedures are oral and public and no expert-witness can take the stand without stating his qualifications, training and experience. He is faced with an examination-in-chief, cross-examination and he must be well prepared. His task is alleviated by the fact that he can use his notes when he testifies. That is not allowed to the expert-witness in the civil law tradition. He has to take the stand without notes and he has to remember every fact by heart.

Court-appointed experts or assessors can be appointed in common law countries, but this is not often done and even contested. The main reason why courts shall not appoint an expert of the court is: 'the presence of a court-sponsored witness, who would most certainly create a strong, if not overwhelming impression of *impartiality* and *objectivity*, could potentially transform a trial by jury into a trial by witnesses.

The chain of evidence

Whenever an expert receives a piece of evidence to investigate, he is responsible for that evidence and he has to make sure that the evidence will not be destroyed, deformed, lost or damaged. There is no substantial difference in the way common law and civil law legislation handle these cases. The fact that evidence may not be destroyed or damaged does not mean that the expert may not touch or investigate the pieces of evidence. He would otherwise be unable to perform his mission. All he has to do is to make a report or to keep a worksheet that gives all the details of the performed investigation, the dates and the hours that the pieces of evidence were handled and the nature of the investigation.

If a forensic odontologist receives a skull to perform age estimation, he will take out a couple of teeth, which subsequently are prepared and slices are made. That means that these teeth are destroyed for the investigation, but there is no other way of doing it. The only thing he has to do is to make sure that the used pieces of teeth remain with the skull.

If the experts asks the assistance of another colleague or another specialist, he has to make sure that he is supervising the work done by his colleague and that the evidence does not slip from his hands. This uninterrupted chain of evidence has attracted a lot of importance in common law jurisdictions lately. In civil law jurisdictions, the report of the expert must contain a description of the exact evolution of the forensic work performed and the statements in that report about the chronological tasks performed are presumed to be absolutely true, unless it can be proven otherwise.

The burden of proof that the chain of evidence is broken, that the reliability of the evidence is jeopardised is on the defense.

Civil and criminal liability of expert-witnesses

On a public policy level, it is likely that the justifications adduced in support of witnesses' immunity from negligence suits would not avail in a case where deliberate dishonesty was perpetrated by an expert in the form of a report tendered to the court or in the form of oral testimony.

The likely approach of modern courts is unreceptiveness to the contention that expert-witnesses, purely because of their formal status, should be exempted from criminal liability should there be evidence that they have deliberately attempted to mislead the courts by offering false information or views that they do not hold. But proceedings for perjury will be extremely infrequent because of the enormous difficulties of proof to the criminal standard.

The fact that the expert is cross-examined (at least in common law countries) is another guarantee that false expert's opinions will not be able to decide a case. And, furthermore, each expert knows that his reliability and professional honour or even career is at stake.

However, something of a shift from the generous judicial attitude of the past can be perceived in Palmer vs Dunford Ford, 1992 where judge Tuckey QC said: ' the immunity extended to them for protection from negligence action was based on public policy grounds and so should only be conferred where it is absolutely necessary to do so.

Generally I do not think that liability for failure to give careful advice to his client should inhibit an expert from giving truthful and fair evidence in court...

I can see no good reason why an expert should not be liable for the advice he gives to his client as to the merits of the claim, particularly if proceedings have not yet been started, and a fortiori, as to whether he is qualified to advise at all.

Thus, the immunity would only extend to what could fairly be said to be preliminary to his giving evidence in court judged perhaps by the principal purpose for which the work was done.

So the production or approval of a report for the purposes of disclosure to the other side would be immune but work done for the principal purpose of advising the client would not'.

Confidentiality and the forensic odontologist

Professional confidentiality is a basic duty of the medical practitioner and a fundamental right of the patient. The principle has been laid down in written form in the Oath of Hippocrates, but the meaning has changed over time.

The medical world would not be able to function properly without confidentiality and trust in the medical profession would be non-existent.

In Belgium the rule is laid down in article 458 of the penal code and reads as follows: 'No medical professional can divulge the secrets and confidences of his patients, unless he has to testify in court or when the law obliges him to do so'.

The punishment is an imprisonment of 8 days up to 6 months and a fine of 100 to 500 francs (to be multiplied by 60).

Is this rule absolute, must it be respected in all circumstances? Who decides when the rule can be broken? What does professional confidentiality mean?

Professional confidentiality covers all knowledge:
-    attained during the practice of medicine;
-    with a confidential character;
-    that has been trusted to the practitioner.

An infraction on the rule has to be done 'on purpose'. Generally recognized exceptions to the rule are:
-    giving evidence or testifying in a court of law;
-    producing a medical file upon request of the court;

-    a legal duty such as the declaration of infectious or sexual transmitted diseases or the declaration of birth and death.

When a doctor has to appear in court to testify, he has to appear, he must take the oath, but then he can decide whether he will give the information or not. He cannot be forced to speak up, if he thinks that he has to remain silent. He decides freely and alone, even if he has been dismissed of his duty.

The judge has the opportunity to evaluate, after careful consideration of all the circumstances of the case, that the witness, who refuses to testify, does not divert the professional secret from his aim (Cass. nr.690 dd. 23.09.1986).

The major part of the medical profession in Belgium is of the opinion that the professional confidentiality rule is an absolute one and that even if the patient dismisses the doctor of his duty, he has no right to give any information at all.

If that should be the general rule then the Courts may sometimes have great difficulties in establishing the truth and it is not abnormal that such an attitude is open to criticism. The professional confidentiality rule has two components: there is the public interest that every patient could be sure that his doctor will not divulge the confidences that he has made to him and on the other hand there is the individual interest of the patient who sometimes needs a written statement of his doctor about his health condition to obtain a profit (social or financial).

We have to consider that today the patient does no longer accept the vertical way of care in the doctor-patient relation. The attitude has changed to a horizontal relation in which the patient decides or at least participates actively in the decision making about what shall be done to him.

It would be desirable to see the confidentiality rule as a part of the contractual relation between doctor and patient, and there should be a balance between confidentiality and information, as well as between the deciding power of the doctor and the right to self-determination of the patient.

This would mean that the keeper of the secret (doctor) can no longer withhold information if that information should be in the interest of the one entitled to the secret (patient). That will be the case when moral or even material interests of the patient are at stake: insurances, labor conditions, etc...

What about the confidentiality rule in the case of a battered child, wife, grandpa or grandma, or the handicapped. We know that the rule only works in the doctor-patient relation and not towards third parties. If the culprit has no professional relation with the doctor then he is not bound by the rule and he has a duty to report (Cass. nr.1121 dd. 09.02.1988).

It may be different if the parents of a battered child are also his patients. In that case the rule is working again. A doctor can invoke a state of emergency to break the rule if he has reasons to believe that there was an immediate and serious danger to a person or to the public at large. He then has to consider the respective values of the conflicting duties, before he makes up his mind (Cass. nr.5728 dd. 13.05.1987).

So if the condition of the child is such that immediate danger is present or that the battery went on for a long time he has to take the necessary steps to avoid further damage to the health of his patient. Most of the time the doctor will report to the special centres for child abuse and seldom immediately to the legal authorities.

Another example can be found if a doctor knows that the health condition of one of his patients is such that he is an imminent danger to other persons, for example when he knows that a person can no longer drive a car or conduct a train or bus safely.

The conclusion of this part of the lecture can be that professional confidentiality is a right shared by doctor and patient and that both individual and public interests have to be considered before any decision is made to break the rule or not.

The confidentiality rule and the medical expert-witness

A medical expert-witness is both a doctor and an expert-witness. Does the rule applies? The expert-witness is appointed by a judge of instruction, a magistrate or the court and he has a public mission to fulfil. He is not treating a patient, so there is no doctor-patient relation and consequently no confidentiality rule. That's the main reason why a doctor can never be appointed to be an expert-witness in a case in which one of his patients is involved.

Even if the expert is not bound by the confidentiality rule, we have to consider that:
-       his mission is personal and he cannot disclose any information about it to third parties because the penal procedure is a secret one in the first stage;
-       an investigation and a conclusion, based on documents covered by the professional secret, is invalid;
-       the expert cannot investigate beyond the limits of his mission, but if he thinks that his mission is incomplete and that it is necessary for his investigation to have it enlarged, he can always ask the judge or the magistrate to do so.

A medical expert-witness who wants entry to medical files, which may be covered by the secret, has no right to lay his hand on them or to request that these files should be given to him. He must ask the judge for a court order to make sure that these documents will be added to the file of investigation. It is however possible that the doctor, after consulting his patient, releases the necessary information.

An expert-witness shall before he starts his investigation and when he has to examine a suspect (for example in bite mark cases), make perfectly clear that he is the expert-witness. He shall communicate the content of his mission, what kind of investigations he will do and what will be done with it. So the suspect knows that the expert-witness is not bound by the secret, if he sticks within the limits of his mission.

A difficult problem may arise when the suspect admits the crime in front of the medical expert-witness during the investigation. What then about the confidentiality rule? Most authors think that the medical doctor has been appointed to fulfil his mission and that such confidences do not change his mission. Solving the crime is work for the police and the legal authorities. But we have seen before that a doctor can invoke a state of emergency to break the rule if he has reasons to believe that there was an immediate and serious danger to a person or to the public at large. He then has to consider the respective values of the conflicting duties, before he makes up his mind (Cass. nr.5728 dd. 13.05.1987).

An expert-witness is not bound by the professional secret, as long as he stays within the limits of his mission. Beyond this mission he has to remain silent, unless some higher values have to be protected.

How reliable is our dental age estimation?

The impact of diet on age at death determinations based on molar attrition

G.J.R. Maat

LEIDEN UNIVERSITY - THE NETHERLANDS
FACULTY OF MEDICINE
DEPARTMENT OF ANATOMY AND EMBRYOLOGY

Introduction

Since many years Don Brothwell's method for age at death determination is the most popular and widespread amongst methods based on molar attrition (Brothwell, 1972). With the help of his classification the degree of molar attrition i.e., the pattern of enamel wear and exposed dentine at the occlusal surface, can be easily scored of each molar with the naked eye (Fig. 1). For subsequent age at death diagnosis the interrelated scores of the juxtapositioned first, second and third molar can be directly coupled with a certain age at death interval in his age-attrition table (Fig. 2). But one has to realize that this method was based on and was meant for Pre-Mediaeval West-European populations. Due to cultural evolution and improvements in food processing the coarseness of the diet and thus the rate of molar attrition changed (decreased) with time. Consequently age-attrition tables have to be adapted. To elucitate the impact of diet on age at death

determinations based on molar attrition a comparison was made between a Pre-
Mediaeval (British), a Late Mediaeval (Dutch) and a 17-18th century (Dutch)
West-European population.

FIG. 1.   NUMERICAL CLASSIFICATION OF MOLAR ATTRITION. Modified from Brothwell, 1972.

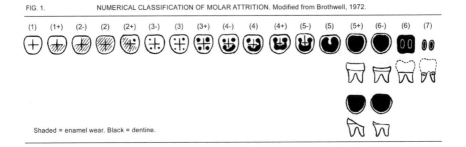

Shaded = enamel wear. Black = dentine.

Materials and methods

The British material investigated by Brothwell (1972) consisted of an
unknown number of specimens dating from the Neolithic (4000 BC) to Mediaeval
Period. Ages at death of the related individuals were given by ageing status of the
pubic symphyseal face. The Late Mediaeval Dutch material consisted of the
dentitions of 76 citizens buried during 1275-1575 in a churchyard of a Fransiscan
friary in the City of Dordrecht (Maat et al., 1998). The 17-18th century material
was composed of the complete dentitions of 45 Dutch whalers buried on
Spitsbergen (Maat and Van der Velde, 1987). In the latter two samples sex and
skeletal ages at death were determined according to the Workshop of European
Anthropologists (1980).

In all dentitions the molar attrition was scored according to Brothwell
(1972) and Maat and Van Der Velde (1987). M1, M2 and M3 stand for the 'first',
'second' and 'third molar'. The numerical classification of molar wear has an
ordinal interval scale from 1 (no wear) to 7 (only roots left over). The attrition on
the most intact side of the mouth was recorded. On that side all maxillary and
mandibular molars were scored to achieve a mean for M1, M2 and M3. Data were
only eliminated from calculations in case of atypical wear patterns. Means were
compared with Student's t test for paired observations. Regression analysis was
done using the simple linear regression model.

Results

After computing the recorded scores the results from the linear regression
model were displayed in a similar way as originally done by Brothwell in his age-
attrition table (1972). They can be found in the Figures 2, 3 and 4.

In the Pre-Mediaeval Period the degree of attrition increased gradually from 3(M1), 2+(M2), 1(M3) for the 17-25 years age interval to any greater degree than 5+(M1), 5(M2), 4+(M3) for the 45+ (plus) age interval.

In the Late Mediaeval Period the degree of attrition increased from 3-(M1), 2-/2(M3), 1+(M1) for the 14-17 years age interval to 5-/5(M1), 4(M2), 3+(M3) for the 65-70+ (plus) interval.

In the 17-18th century the degree of attrition increased from 2+(M1), 1+/2-(M2), 1(M3) for the 14-17 years age interval to 5-(M1), 4-/4(M2), 3/3+(M3) for the 65-70+ (plus) age interval.

FIG. 4   MOLAR ATTRITION DURING THE PERIOD ca. 1650 - 1800 AD[1]

AGE INTERVAL (years)[2]	14 - 17			17 - 25			25 - 35			35 - 45			45 - 55			55 - 65			65 - 70+		
MOLAR	M1	M2	M3	M1	M2	M3	M1	M2	M3	M1	M2	M3	M1	M2	M3	M1	M2	M3	M1	M2	M3
NUMERICAL CLASSIFICATION	2+	1+/2-	1	2+/3-	2	1/1+	3-/3	2/2+	2-/2	3+/4-	2+/3-	2/2+	3+/4-	2+/3-	2+	4-	3-/3	2+/3+	5-	4-/4	3/3+
WEAR PATTERN																					

[1] Scored according to Brothwell (1972) and Maat and van der Velde (1987). N = 45 whalers with complete dentitions buried on Spitsbergen (Maat and van der Velde, 1987).
[2] Ages are skeletal ages assessed according to the WEA (1980).

Fig. 2   MOLAR ATTRITION DURING THE PRE-MEDIAEVAL PERIOD (Brothwell, 1972)[1]

AGE INTERVAL (years)[2]	17 - 25			25 - 35			35 - 45			45+		
MOLAR	M1	M2	M3	M1	M2	M3	M1	M2	M3	M1	M2	M3
NUMERICAL CLASSIFICATION	3	2+	1	4+	4-	3-	5+	5	4+	Any greater degree		
WEAR PATTERN										Any greater degree		

[1] Modified from Brothwell (1972), and scored according to Maat and van der Velde (1987). Several early British groups.
[2] Ages are skeletal ages assessed by the pubic symphyseal face.

FIG. 3   MOLAR ATTRITION DURING THE PERIOD ca. 1275 - 1572, AD[1]

AGE INTERVAL (years)[2]	14 - 17			17 - 25			25 - 35			35 - 45			45 - 55			55 - 65			65 - 70+		
MOLAR	M1	M2	M3	M1	M2	M3	M1	M2	M3	M1	M2	M3	M1	M2	M3	M1	M2	M3	M1	M2	M3
NUMERICAL CLASSIFICATION	3-	2-/2	1+	3-/3	2	1+/2-	3/3+	2+/3-	2-/2	4-	3-/3	2/2+	4	3/3+	2+/3-	4+/5-	4-	3	5-/5	4	3+
WEAR PATTERN																					

[1] Scored according to Brothwell (1972) and Maat and van der Velde (1987). N = 76 citizens buried in a churchyard of a Fransiscan friary in the City of Dordrecht.
[2] Ages are skeletal ages assessed according to the WEA (1980).

Discussion

After comparison of the three diagrams (Figs. 2-4) it is clear that in western Europe the rate of molar attrition decreased dramatically during the time span covered by the three samples. The average wear pattern as for instance seen in the 35-45 age interval during the Pre-Mediaeval Period was never accomplished during later periods, not even by individuals of the oldest age at death interval (i.e., 65-70+ years). The average wear pattern as seen in the 25-35 age interval during the Pre-Mediaeval Period was only accomplished in the 55-65 age interval of the Late Mediaeval Period and in the 65-70+ age interval of the 17-18th century. If compared to the Pre-Mediaeval Period the latter two shifts in functional age of teeth represented about 30 and 40 years respectively! Most likely these shifts were the result of a substantial decrease in coarseness of foodstuffs in the diet. For instance it is known that during the transition from the Mediaeval Period to the 17-18th century grain millers started to bolt flour through fine cloth sieves to remove coarse particles of bran (Burema, 1953; Moore and Corbett, 1975). As a result the overall rate of attrition will have decreased considerably in the population. If so, then as a matter of course, the impact of diet has to be taken into consideration when applying age at death determination methods based on molar attrition. The best way to do so is by making a specific reference age-attrition table by means of seriation of dentitions of individuals of documented/skeletal- age from a particular cultural or time period.

The results strongly suggest that molar attrition can only be used as an age at death indicator if its application is restricted to a particular cultural period and diet.

Summary

To elucidate the impact of diet on age at death determinations based on molar attrition a comparison was made between the rate of attrition in a Pre-Mediaeval (British), a Late Mediaeval (Dutch) and a 17-18th century (Dutch) West-European population. It appeared that the rate decreased dramatically during that time span. Most likely this change was diet related i.e., to the coarsness of foodstuffs. This result strongly indicates that molar attrition can only be used as an age at death indicator if its application is restricted to a particular cultural period and diet.

References

Brothwell D.R. (1972) Digging up bones. British Museum, London.

Burema L. (1953) De voeding in Nederland van de Middeleeuwen tot de twintigste eeuw. Van Gorkum, Assen.

Maat G.J.R. and Van der Velde E.A. (1987) The caries attrition competition. *International Journal of Anthropology* **2**: 281-292.

Maat G.J.R., Mastwijk R.W., Sarfatij H. (1998) A physical anthropological study of burials from the graveyard of the Fransiscan Friary at Dordrecht (circa 1275-1572 AD). State Service for Archeological Investigations in The Netherlands (ROB), Amersfoort. *Rapporten Archeologische Monumentenzorg* **67**: 46.

Moore W.J. and Corbett M.E. (1975). Distribution of dental caries in ancient British populations. III. The 17th century. *Caries Research* **9**: 163-175.

Workshop of European Anthropologists. (1980) Recommendations for age and sex diagnosis of skeletons. *Journal of Human Evolution* **9**: 517-549.

A correlation between dental age and bone age

V.M. Phillips and I.O.C. Thompson

University Stellenbosch - South Africa
Department of Oral Pathology

Introduction

The forensic dentist may utilize a hand-wrist radiograph to assess the skeletal age of children of similar genetic constitutions and similar socio-economic circumstances. These radiographs provide detailed information about the growth progress of the individual towards maturity. They permit the assessment of maturation rates of the individual shafted (long) and non-shafted (round or irregular) bones. The initial appearance of each bone's ossification centre(s) reflects the stage of development of the skeletal system and relates to the physiological age of the individual. These maturity indicators also show the relative developmental precocity of the female compared to the male. Most children develop at different rates because of genetic differences even when adequately nourished. There are, however, early and late maturing children. There are also racial differences in skeletal developmental rates among different populations. There remains a lack of information with regard to environmental factors affecting the growth and development of children as related to their skeletal and dental development. Greulich and Pyle (1959) published male and female hand-wrist film standards for white children from Cleveland and Boston. In the utilization of the hand-wrist radiograph the observer must be familiar with the appearance of maturity indicators. The 30 bones of the hand and wrist are preformed in cartilage and develop endochondrally. The ossification centres in the shafted bones appear prenatal. The epiphyses' ossification centres in shafted and non-shafted bones appear in an orderly sequence. There are, however, irregularities in the order of ossification.

The basal bone of the maxilla and mandible grows and matures at the same rate as the appendicular skeleton. Terminal growth of the mandible and some calvarial bones are prolonged and mature at the age of approximately 30 to 40 years. The transitional features of the growing hand and wrist-bones do not correlate well with dental maturation or eruption sequences.

Age determination by means of the teeth is well documented and a relatively reliable means of assessing the age of a young individual. The most extensive research in this field was done by Nolla (1960), Moorrees et al. (1963) and Gustafson (1966) where the development and calcification of the crowns and roots of the teeth were related to the chronological age of European and American individuals. Altini (1983) undertook a preliminary investigation to produce a regression curve applicable to black South Africans. This showed a significant difference to the regression curve for Europeans as published by Gustafson (1966). The mesial root of the 3rd molar was investigated by Harris and Nortje (1984) and reviewed by Van Heerden (1989). These authors suggest that the third molar tooth development provided a valuable aid to the assessment of chronological age between the ages of 14 and 21 years.

Recently there have been a series of severely decomposed bodies of 22 children and young adults found on the Cape Flats in the Western Cape Province. These have been linked to a serial killer that sodomised his victims and then strangulated them. All of these victims have been buried face down in a partially clothed state. During the post-mortem procedures, identification of these victims was of prime importance and the age estimation of these children was an important factor. Tables of the calcification stages of the teeth published by Moorrees et al. (1963), Schour and Massler (1941) were used to estimate the ages of some of these victims. Most of these victims had no dental records and few had had any dental treatment other than the removal of carious deciduous teeth. Most of the victims were identified by means of their clothing, but the clothes of those in which advanced decomposition had taken place were of little help. Age estimation became an important factor in the identification of these children. The results of this investigation led the authors to doubt the efficacy of the published tables for age estimation on this population group. A pilot study was undertaken to compare the dental and skeletal ages of a sample of the South African population in the Western Cape.

Materials and methods

Pantomographic radiographs of the jaws and hand-wrist radiographs of children of 3 racial groups were obtained from the Orthodontic Department of the Dental Faculty of the University of Stellenbosch. The skeletal ages of the children were estimated using the figures of Greulich and Pyle (1959). The dental ages were estimated using the figures of Morrees et al. (1963). The sample consisted of 86 Caucasians (42M, 44F), 89 mixed racial group (35M, 54F), and 14 Negroid (3M, 11F) children. The age range of the children was from 2 to 21 years. The estimated dental and skeletal ages were correlated with the chronological age of each child and the results were analyzed.

Results

The average dental age estimation for the Caucasian children under-estimated their ages by 0.5 years (SD=1.36), the Mixed group ages were under-estimated by 0.1 years (SD=1.63) and the Negroid group ages were over-estimated by 1.0 year (SD=1.80).

The average skeletal ages of the children from the Caucasian, Negroid and Mixed groups were under-estimated by 1.0 year (SD=1.80).

Conclusion

The skeletal age estimation of a sample of South African children showed an average under-estimation of their ages by approximately 1 year. The dental age estimation was more accurate for the children of mixed origin than it was for children of the other two race groups. The dental age estimation for Caucasian children was marginally more accurate than the skeletal estimation, but the age estimation for Negroid children using either teeth or bones were equally inaccurate

This pilot study indicates that a wider study is necessary to establish a database for the skeletal and dental age estimation of South African children from all race groups.

References

Altini M. (1983) Age determination from the teeth. *Journal of the Dental Association South Africa* **38**: 275-279.

Greulich W.W. and Pyle S.I. (1959) Radiographic atlas of skeletal development of the hand and wrist. Stanford University Press, Stanford, California.

Gustafson G. (1966) Forensic odontology. Staples Press, London, United Kingdom, p102-108.

Harris M.J.P. and Nortje C.J. (1984) The mesial root of the third molar: a possible indicator of age. *Journal of Forensic Odonto-Stomatology* **2**: 39-43.

Moorrees C.F.A., Fanning E.A., Hunt E.E. (1963) Age variation of formation stages for ten permanent teeth. *Journal of Dental Research* **42**: 1490-1502.

Nolla C.M. (1960) The development of the permanent teeth. *Journal of Dentistry for Children* **27**: 254-266.

Schour I. and Massler M. (1941) The development of the human dentition. *Journal of the American Dental Association* **20**: 379-427.

Van Heerden P.J. (1985) The mesial root of the third mandibular molar as a possible indicator of age. Dissertation for Diploma in Forensic Odontology, London Hospital Medical College, London, United Kingdom.

Age estimation in adults

T. Solheim* and S. Kvaal

UNIVERSITY OF OSLO - NORWAY
FACULTY OF DENTISTRY
DEPARTMENT OF ORAL PATHOLOGY AND FORENSIC ODONTOLOGY

Introduction

Estimation of the age of individuals dead or alive may be of importance in a number of situations. In living persons the reason may be that the person has lost his memory or the age is unknown such as in refugees or adopted children. Sometimes the police may have a suspicion that the age has been falsified for some reason. Also the involved person may claim that his date of birth was not correctly registered as he entered the country and wants it changed. Often children are involved, but also it may also be adults. The accuracy of any method is much better in children than adults where any estimate may fail a lot.

In dead persons estimation of age may be of importance when the identity is unknown. Even when the police have some indication of the identity an estimate of the age may be used as evidence for the identity if other evidence is weak. However, in a case where the identity is totally unknown age estimates may be of utmost importance in the reconstruction of the identity. When only the skeleton is left from an individual, age estimation may be even more important in the reconstructive identification. This may be especially so in archaeological materials.

Anthropologists may estimate the age from the state of closure of the bone sutures and epiphyseal plates. The same may be used in living persons where physicians from radiographs may assess the state of closure.

Anthropologists usually rely on the closure of sutures etc but may also use the state of dental attrition as a bases for their estimates of age. Seldom are specific dental methods used as opposed to in forensic medicine where consulting forensic odontologists have a number of methods available for their use.

History

Early methods of age estimation have been just a visual estimate. It has been shown that experienced dentists may give a quite reliable estimate of the age of a person based on the teeth only (Solheim and Sundnes, 1980). Also old horse traders used the teeth to assess the age of a horse they wanted to buy.

Gustafson's method

A more scientific method was introduced by the Swedish professor in oral pathology, professor Gøsta Gustafson in 1947 (Gustafson, 1947) and published in English in 1950 (Gustafson, 1950). He used 4 scores (0,1,2,3) of the various age changes such as attrition, periodontal recession, secondary dentin formation, apical translucency, apical resorption and cementum apposition. The scores were added up and a regression analysis made with sum of scores as independent variable and age as dependent variable.

Newer morphologic methods

Despite statistical difficulties this method gained wide acceptance and still today may be the method of choice, especially in America. However, a number of attempts have been made to set up a better method. The first was Dalitz from Melbourne Australia (1962) who used computerised multiple regression. In addition, he increased the number of scores to 5 and omitted the resorption and cementum apposition as being too weakly related to the age. Gunnar Johanson (1971) increased the number of scores to 7 and also used multiple regression. It is sure (possible) that these authors used more than one tooth from the same individual and as the formula did not differentiate between different types of teeth, the statistics would be incorrect.

A further improvement came with Maples (1978) who introduced tooth position correction factors. His number of scores were however only 4 as he did not know the works of Dalitz nor Johanson.

Solheim (1993) published a method based on a large number of teeth and on improved statistical principles and we will later introduce this morphologic method more in detail.

Alternative methods

There has always been a search for simple alternative methods that might even be more reliable. Also the need to grind the tooth may not be acceptable if the material should be preserved. One of the first to present such a method was Bang and Ramm (1970) and it was based on the length of the translucent zone only and special formulas were developed both for sectioned and for unsectioned teeth.

A method based on the colour as the only criterion has also been introduced (Ten Cate et al., 1977). The colour has been shown to reflect the age well and was also included in the morphologic method (Solheim, 1993).

Internal changes in teeth can be studied in radiographs. A method based on radiographs, but unfortunately trying to apply Gustafson's scores, was presented (Matsikidis and Schulz, 1982). This method was further elaborated by Kvaal and Solheim (1994). Also a more extensive method based on radiographs only have been presented as a radiographic method and will be further discussed later (Kvaal et al., 1995).

Other methods that have been claimed to be accurate is the counting of cementum annulation rings (Grosskopf, 1990). After an extensive investigation we found that that method may be fairly accurate only up to about 30 years in human. After that the accuracy is much reduced with increasing age (Kvaal and Solheim, 1995).

A method based on the rasemization of aminoacids like aspartic acid has been considered to be biologic chronometer (Ritz et al., 1993). It has been shown to have a correlation with age between 0.95 and 0.99 (Mörnstad et al., 1994).

Age estimation in adults

As the statistical variation in the accuracy is not impressive with a standard deviation of about 10 years, any technique will occasionally give aberrant results. Also a visual estimate from a single tooth by an experienced dentist may not be so much more incorrect (Solheim and Sundnes, 1980). In fact, when employing the whole dentition in a case a dentist may often perform better than the more scientific statistical methods.

For practical purposes in age estimation cases it is recommended that the expert first estimates the age after a visual assessment of the whole dentition. Then the method(s) of choice in the case and according to the circumstances should be selected. If possible, more than one statistical method should be used. If one method fails severely, the other may give a more correct result. A prerequisite for this quality control is that the two different methods are using different parameters. The obtained results should be compared with the original visual assessment, and the expert should have so much self-confidence that he lets his own estimate count heavily for the final estimate.

Recommended statistical methods

The method of Bang (1970)

This is a simple method which may be executed on all teeth or tooth roots. It may be done on sectioned teeth, but works generally equally well on unsectioned teeth. The tooth should be held against a good light source, but not so that the eyes of the observer are illuminated. The length of the translucent zone should be measured with a sliding caliper. Here lays the subjectivity of this method as this length is not always well defined and has to be estimated. Especially in sectioned teeth the length may vary from the periphery to the area near the pulp and also on the two sides of the pulp. When the length has been measured the appropriate formula may be used and the value of the constants looked up in the table. Then the age may be calculated. It will improve the reliability to use more than one tooth.

The morphologic method (Solheim 1993)

Even though several morphologic methods have been advised through the years, I of course believe the method I have published in many cases should be the method of choice. It is based on a large material of about 1000 teeth, molars excluded. Left and right teeth are pooled, but only so that only one tooth of each type from each individual was used in the final calculations.

It was the aim to measure the variables instead of scoring them, but the results showed that often the scores were more closely related to age than the measurements. Therefore, scores were used for most changes and two new types of scores were developed.

Also this method is based on sectioned teeth. However, for the maxillary second premolar (15/25) all changes can be measured on the unsectioned tooth. This tooth is therefore used as indicator tooth in cases where one does not want to destroy the tooth. For other cases one or several teeth must be ground to the mid-pulpal area (Solheim, 1984). Alternative formulas for unextracted teeth have also been calculated. These are using only the attrition, tooth colour and recession of the periodontal ligament, but the accuracy is of course reduced (Solheim, 1994).

The radiographic method (Kvaal et al., 1995)

This method is based on measurements on radiographs taken in an orthoradial projection. Six teeth have been chosen as indicator teeth after preliminary studies of relationship with age e.g. maxillary 1, 2 and 5 and mandibular 2, 3 and 4. Either left or right teeth may be used.

The principle is that the ratio between pulp length and tooth/root length and also between pulp/root width at the cervical margin and in the mid-root area and midway between these. Formulas are calculated based on multiple regression and either formulas for each tooth or a joint formula for mandibular or maxillary teeth may be used. Also a joint formula for all 6 teeth have been calculated. The latter showed the strongest correlation with age.

Recommendations

The approach to age estimation should vary according to the situation. Obviously, when it is not so important less time should be put into the work. I generally recommend a visual assessment of the age to be made in all post mortem examinations. Be careful to base the assessment on the teeth only. It is tempting to take the general appearance of the person and the skin into consideration. However, this is the responsibility of the forensic pathologist and if the dental evaluation should be a real complementary technique, it should not be based on the same criteria. If you do this it will also give you experience and improve your performance. In fact, an experienced dentist often gives astonishing good visual estimates of the age based on the entire dentition.

If it becomes more important that the estimate you give is as accurate as possible, the visual assessment should be supplemented by one or preferably two different statistical techniques. An important question will then be if one or several teeth can be taken out of the alveole as in dead persons. Obviously, in living persons this can not be done. In these cases the radiographic method will be the method of choice. If you want to employ an alternative method, the morphologic method based only on criteria that can be assessed from unextracted teeth should be used. In dead persons teeth can normally be extracted and even ground to the mid-pulpal area. If you just want a quick check of your visual estimate the translucency method either as described by Bang and Ramm (1970) or by Solheim (1989) should be used. For a more accurate age estimate the use of the morphologic method if possible made on several teeth is recommended. In addition, the radiographic method could be used as a supplement. In dead persons, either in precious archaelogical material or forensic odontological material the teeth should not be extracted only lifted out of the alveole if possible without destruction. In such cases the teeth should certainly not be ground and thus destructed. In these cases, the radiographic technique should be the method of choice. However, the morphologic technique, especially if the maxillary 5 is available is a good supplement.

References

Bang G. and Ramm E. (1970) Determination of age in humans from root dentin transparency. *Acta Odontologica Scandinavica* **28**: 3-35.

Dalitz G.D. (1962) Age determination of adult human remains by teeth examination. *Journal of the Forensic Science Society* **3**: 11-21.

Grosskopf B. (1990) Individualaltersbestimmung mit Hilfe von Zuwachsringen im Zement bodengelagerter menschlicher Zähne. (Individual age determination using growth rings in the cementum of buried human teeth). *Zeitschrift für Rechtsmedizin* **103**: 351-359.

Gustafson G. (1947) Åldersbestämningar på tänder. *Odontologisk Tidskrift* **55**: 556-568.

Gustafson G. (1950) Age determination on teeth. *Journal of the American Dental Association* **41**: 45-54.

Johanson G. (1971) Age determination from teeth. *Odontologisk Revy* **22**: 1-126.

Kvaal S.I. and Solheim T. (1994) A non-destructive dental method for age estimation. *Journal of Forensic Odonto-Stomatology* **12**: 6-11.

Kvaal S.I. and Solheim T. (1995) Incremental lines in human dental cementum in relation to age. *European Journal of Oral Science* **103**: 225-230.

Kvaal S.I., Kolltveit K.M., Thompsen I.O., Solheim T. (1995) Age estimation of adults from dental radiographs. *Forensic Science International* **74**: 175-185.

Maples W.R. (1978) An improved technique using dental histology for estimation of adult age. *Journal of Forensic Sciences* **23**: 764-770.

Matsikidis G. and Schulz P. (1982) Altersbestimmung nach dem Gebiss mit Hilfe des Zahnfilms. (Age determination by dentition with the aid of dental films). *Zahnärztliche Mitteilungen* **72**: 2524-2528.

Mörnstad H., Pfeiffer H., Teivens A. (1994) Estimation of dental age using HPLC-technique to determine the degree of aspartic acid racemization. *Journal of Forensic Sciences* **39**: 1425-1431.

Ritz S., Schutz H.W., Peper C. (1993) Post mortem estimation of age at death based on aspartic acid racemization in dentin. Its application for root dentin. *International Journal of Legal Medicine* **105**: 289-293.

Solheim T. (1984) Dental age estimation. An alternative technique for tooth sectioning. *American Journal of Forensic Medicine and Pathology* **5**: 181-184.

Solheim T. (1989) Dental root translucency as an indicator of age. *Scandinavian Journal of Dental Research* **97**: 189-197.

Solheim T. (1993) A new method for dental age estimation in adults. *Forensic Science International* **59**: 137-147.

Solheim T. (1994) En ny metode for å beregne alderen hos voksne basert på ikke-ekstraherte tenner. In: Kongressrapport. XII Nordiske MØte I Rettsmedisin. *Nordic Society of Forensic Medicine Proceedings* pp. 72-76.

Solheim T. and Sundnes P.K. (1980) Dental age estimation of Norwegian adults - a comparison of different methods. *Forensic Science International* **16**: 7-17.

Ten Cate A.R., Thompson G.W., Dickinson J.B., Hunter H.A. (1977) The estimation of age of skeletal remains from the colour of roots of teeth. *Canadian Dental Association Journal* **43**: 83-86.

Identification and use of probabilities in forensic odontology

A philosophical discussion

F. Taroni

Université de Lausanne - Switzerland
Institut Universitaire de Médecine Légale

Courts are showing more and more circumspection when dealing with scientific evidence interpretation. This debate (on the way of presenting evidence) became apparent during experts' testimonies on DNA genetic evidence and could well extend to all forensic science disciplines. Despite half a century of practice vouching for its qualities, dentistry will not escape questioning as far as the scientific interpretation of evidence is concerned.

To a sensible observer considering evidence investigation practices in dentistry (for instance, the link existing between a bite mark and the dentition of a suspect), the conflicts of opinion(s) observed among practitioners world-wide can easily give rise to doubts on the foundations of the science.

Many experts consider a minimal number of characteristics: a formal identification is established only if the minimal number of corresponding characteristics between the observed mark and the picture of the set of teeth or dentures from the potential source of the mark is put in evidence and no unexplained unconformity is observed.

Other experts exclude the idea of a minimum numerical standard. For them identification is a matter of judgement/good sense. The expert evaluates the contributions to individuality on a quantitative (number of characteristics) and a qualitative (peculiar characteristics, mark clearness, etc.) level.

Most experts refuse to give advisable opinion(s) (including experts in dactyloscopy, a science which inspired evidence interpretation in dentistry) pronouncing themselves either for an identification or an exclusion (except occasionally when no decision can be reached). They thus favour a deterministic approach to the detriment of a probabilistic one. This means in practice that a mark presenting 5 characteristics for example in common with a potential source may, in the end, have no conclusive value depending on the approach chosen.

This leading article questions the practitioners' deterministic approach(es) and notes the limits of their conclusions in order to encourage a discussion to question current practices. With this end in view, a hypothetical discussion between an expert in dentistry and an enthousiastic member of a jury, eager to understand the scientific principles of evidence interpretation, is presented. This discussion will lead us to regard any argument aiming at identification as probabilistic.

During this debate, our two protagonists will be joined by a judge to remind us of the expert's precious help in the hands of Justice, which allows the judge, as a last resort, to act as a moral certainty on the analysed facts.

Now let our protagonists speak:

Juror: In order to clear up my mind and better interpret the conclusions of your report, I would like to start with a preliminary question about numerical standards. Are the decisions, which have been taken towards a minimum numerical standard, based on scientific results or do they rather fulfil mandatory practices?

Expert: I must say, that as far as identification is concerned no theory can justify a fixed numerical standard (Champod, 1996). The identification process required goes beyond a mere counting of characteristics.

Juror: Therefore I do not understand all the reticence towards qualified advice in dentistry.

Expert: It seems impossible that the notion of probability can be applied to evidence. Experts have argued that every single tiny part of the tooth surface is strictly individual. The hypothesis that a mark could have several donors thus appears inconceivable.

Juror: I think I understand your argument. The information given by each part of the dental surface is complete and individual. However, can you say as much for fragmentary or ill-printed marks? In case of a transferred mark, how do you explain the differences of interpretation methods between the mark and other comparable ones such as biological evidence (blood, sperm, etc.)? Is not any biological fluid also strictly specific to an individual when the DNA molecule is exhaustively studied? Qualified advice, i.e. the capacity to give an opinion combined to a probability seems to be an easy task for experts in genetics. So where does all this reticence come from? Does not the acceptance of qualified advice mean a questioning of the very concept(s) of identification?

Expert: Careful! Even if we accept your argument, the absence of figures could well make experts reticent when it comes to probabilities. The provision of qualified advice implies that the expert is also able to estimate the probability of the trace in question (or the number of persons that could be taken into account as being potential suspects). However, statistical data on variability are not numerous, not to say non-existent, when compared to the individuality which results from the combination of numerous factors, such as the general dental shape, outline of the characteristics, for example.

Juror: If I understand you correctly, the aim is thus to collect statistical data and determine a model to estimate the probability of the shape of a dental characteristic. This seems logical and conforms with Locard's doctrine on fingerprints applied to the rules of the identification process. He wrote notably: «there are few characteristics: in that case (the) print(s) show(s) no certainty but a presumption proportional to the number of points and their sharpness» (Locard, 1914). Locard considered that there was more to the evaluation of an identification than a mere counting of characteristics.

Expert: Exactly. It is erroneous to regard scientific evidence as dichotomous asserting only an identification or an exclusion. Given the increasing set of values between exclusion and identification such a sharp interpretation appears rather inconceivable.

Juror: Would it therefore be reasonable to think that dental characteristics could evolve by a mere phenomenon of transfer towards «more general» characteristics? For instance, a perfectly sharp break observed directly on a tooth can be regarded as unique. However, if the same break is transferred by pressure on a surface it can, when being taken, look blurred and merge into other dental patterns.

Expert: Yes, the idea of transfer implies necessarily a loss of information and from that moment on, the idea of «more general» characteristics is thoroughly justified. The concept covers a continuum of values, which goes from (a) «poorly/weakly descriptive» to (b) «highly descriptive» characteristic(s).

Juror: ... however judges expect scientific evidence to be one-to-one and
            without any compromise!
Judge: Actually, although judges prefer indisputable evidence, no doubt that
            they would use wisely evidence which without verging on certainty,
            would become integrated into a body of proof. It is worth remembering
            that the expert only brings an element of proof to Court that becomes
            integrated into a body of proof useful for the identification decision.
Expert: Then, the query about « identification » must be regarded as one for the
            judge(s) or Court and not for the expert. In his statement/conclusion(s)
            the expert will just comment on the strength of the link between a mark
            and a tooth where the probability of casual coincidence reaches almost
            0 when it comes to identification.
Judge: At Court, the identification of an individual remains a judiciary matter
            which calls for a group of complicated and ill-matched/dissimilar data,
            as, for instance, material elements, testimonies or other circumstantial
            evidence.

        Although it is not always clearly admitted, the burden of decision rests
with the Court and not with the expert.
        What appears clear is the need:
   -    to emphasise that an element of scientific proof provided by the expert
        is an element among others which aims at supporting (or not) the
        hypothesis of an identification, or more generally, at supporting (or
        not) the link between the mark discovered and a potential donor;
   -    to regard considering the objective part of this type of proof the
        argument proposed by the expert as probabilistic, in the sense that
        from the characteristics observed on the mark he will exclude a certain
        population (to have caused it) and this argument will have to be
        integrated in the Court process of decision (Aitken and MacDonald,
        1979);
   -    to require that from now on efforts be made in the collection of data
        and the application of a model to describe the decision process. One of
        the pioneers of modern criminalistics Kirk already addressed this issue
        in 1964 «Much of this problem [most 'expert testimony' is purely
        opinion testimony] would be avoided if systematic study were devoted
        to the development of sound probability considerations applied to
        evidence interpretation and also to the areas in which statistical
        analysis could properly contribute to correct evaluations. This is a
        field for combined effort by the mathematician and the criminalist. It
        should prove to be a most fruitful area for research – one that would
        strengthen the theoretical foundation on which the more practical
        technical structure could rest with confidence». Reutoul and Smith
        (1973), also have already considered such a questioning/answering

practice: «If it can be stated that they are due to a human bite and they show shapes which an experienced dentist can identify as having been caused by an unusual mouth pattern and there is a suspect who has that pattern then there is a probability that the bites have been caused by the suspect. The degree of probability will depend on the features of the mouth pattern and on how many of these have been transferred to the body. It is here that the evidence of the dentist becomes vital and it is also the position where the forensic medicine expert cannot give a valuable opinion. There does, however, appear to be some conflict of dental opinion on this matter. Perhaps somebody will eventually work out the mathematics of the probability involved. I believe it is necessary to render our methods more efficient by taking greater cognisance of the logical steps in our schemes of identification and not to become lost in the beauty of our instrumentation». Let's just retake and follow their advice.

References

Champod C. (1996) Reconnaissance automatique et analyse statistique des minuties sur les empreintes digitales. Concise: Imprimérie Evard, France.

Locard E. (1914) La preuve judiciaire par les empreintes digitales. *Archives d'anthropologie criminelle, de médecine légale et de psychologie normale et pathologique* **28**: 321-348.

Aitken C.G. and MacDonald D.G. (1979) An application of discrete kernel methods to forensic odontology. *Applied Statistics* **28**: 55-61.

Kirk P.L. (1964) The ontogeny of criminalistics. *The Journal of Criminal Law, Criminology and Police Science* **54**: 235-238.

Reutoul E., Smith H. (1973) Glaister's Medical Jurisprudence and Toxicology. 13th Edn. Edinburgh, Churchill Livingstone, United Kingdom, p66-68.

Teeth, bite marks and DNA

Human bite mark evidence

D. Sweet

UNIVERSITY OF BRITISCH COLUMBIA - CANADA
BUREAU OF LEGAL DENTISTRY (BOLD)

Introduction

The use of bite mark evidence in criminal cases has been widely accepted by law enforcement agencies and courts for many years. Human bite marks can be found on both living and deceased persons. The person may be the victim of a crime. The bite mark may also be found on the perpetrator of a crime because the victim of the attack may use their teeth as a weapon of self-defense. In some cases, non-human bite marks must be examined. For example, animal bites may initially be thought to be human, but a forensic odontologist can usually distinguish between human and animal bites based on the pattern and number of individual teeth. In other cases, inanimate objects, such as foods, coffee cups, chewing gum, pencils, cigarette butts, or other items of physical evidence discovered at the crime scene, are found to contain the imprints of teeth. These can also be investigated in an attempt to identify whose teeth caused the marks.

The crimes in which bite marks may be found include murders, assaults of a sexual or non-sexual nature, homosexual attacks, or cases of physical and sexual abuse. Sexually oriented bite marks are often sadistic in nature and may have been inflicted slowly and deliberately with suction applied to the tissue. Bite marks found in cases of abuse often indicate the rage that is directed against the victim.

Exhibits recovered from victim

Photographs and impressions of the bite marks can be recorded either at the scene of the crime, in the hospital, or in the morgue in the case of a deceased victim. Photographic evidence should depict the bite mark in relation to other anatomical areas (orientation photographs) as well as close-up views with and without a reference scale (ruler). The ABFO No. 2 reference scale, which is an L-shaped millimetre ruler, is widely used. If it is included in the photograph, measurements can be taken of injuries depicted by the photograph, and accurate enlargements of the photograph made, such as life-sized or twice life-sized images.

Saliva washings were taken in the past to attempt to identify the ABO blood group of the perpetrator since 80–85% of humans secrete this information in their saliva. However, more recently, Dr. Sweet has developed methods that make it possible to collect cells from the saliva deposited on the skin during biting, kissing or sucking. Thus, the DNA of the perpetrator can be identified through PCR-based typing of the genetic fingerprint.

The forensic pathologist or forensic odontologist sometimes takes skin sections in an attempt to establish the age of any bruises found in the bite area. The age of the injury is important in order to show that there is in fact an association between the bite mark and the time frame of the crime. Also, through transillumination studies, it may be possible to increase the amount of information available from bruising that is present in the deeper layers of the skin, although individual and accidental dental characteristics (necessary for physical identification) are usually not visible with this technique.

Recovery of exemplars from suspect(s)

In most cases it is easy to collect evidence of the bite injury from the victim. However, to complete a comparison with the teeth of a suspect two things must happen. Firstly, a suspect must be identified and apprehended. Despite many hours of hard work by police agencies, suspects are often not apprehended. Secondly, the suspect must consent to allow evidence such as dental impressions, saliva swabs, and photographs of his teeth to be taken. Alternatively, the criminal code must allow for provision of a warrant to seize this type of evidence from the suspect. In Canada and the United States, laws exist that allow investigators to obtain such warrants providing there is sufficient evidence to suggest that the suspect had some role in the crime (probable cause). The provision of warrants to seize evidence from suspects in other countries varies according to the jurisdiction.

If the suspect agrees to cooperate with the investigation or is compelled to do so through a warrant to seize the exemplars, a complete dental examination of his teeth and mandibular articulation (occlusion and jaw function) is completed. Accurate, full-arch impressions of the upper and lower jaws are taken and study casts are fabricated. An inter-occlusal record to illustrate the relationship of the upper and lower teeth in centric occlusion is also obtained.

Physical comparison of evidence

The evidence collected during this examination is then interpreted and a comparison is made between the dental exemplars from the suspect and the bite mark pattern found in the tissue of the victim. The question to resolve in this comparison, if possible, is whether the bite mark seen on the victim's skin and a test bite mark produced from the suspect's teeth in a material prepared for comparison purposes (such as wax, plasticene, putty, or styrofoam) have a common origin.

One of the most common methods to allow this comparison is to produce a representation of the biting edges of the teeth of interest on a sheet of clear acetate film. Usually the perimeter of the biting edges is recorded to produce an image of each tooth called a hollow volume. The acetate film usually contains life-sized or twice life-sized images of the teeth of interest. The final product is called a hollow volume comparison overlay. Because the biting edges of the teeth are recorded on clear film, the overlay can be superimposed overtop of a similarly enlarged (life-sized or twice life-sized) photograph of the bite mark injury. The overlay can be moved into and out of position while the positions, sizes, shapes of teeth and the configuration and pattern of the dental arches are compared to similar characteristics recorded in the photographic evidence.

Levels of conclusions

Conclusions are reached with respect to how similar or concordant are the teeth and the injuries caused by various teeth depicted in the bite mark. The range of possible conclusions includes a) positive identification, b) probable identification (more likely than not), c) possible identification (cannot exclude), d) insufficient data available (inconclusive), and e) negative identification (exclusion).

Most bite mark evidence is collected and interpreted in order to answer a basic question about a suspect's possible role in the crime: Can the suspect be excluded from the crime? If the forensic odontologist concludes that the suspect's teeth could have caused the bite mark, this information may be used in court to support the theory that the suspect was in violent contact with the victim at the time of the crime.

References

Hernandez-Cueto C., Girela E., Sweet D. J. (2000) Wound vitality diagnosis: a review. *American Journal of Forensic Medicine and Pathology (Accepted)*.

LeRoy H.A. and Sweet D.J. (1993) Take a bite out of crime - Ask a forensic dentist for assistance. *Royal Canadian Mounted Police Gazette* **55**: 1–3.

Pretty I.A., Anderson G.S., Sweet D.J. (1999) Human bites and the risk of HIV infection. *American Journal of Forensic Medicine and Pathology* **20**: 232-239.

Sweet D.J. (1997) Human bite marks: examination, recovery, and analysis. In: Manual of Forensic Odontology - Chapter 5: Bite mark evidence. Bowers C. M. and Bell G. L., eds.. American Society of Forensic Odontology, Colorado Springs, USA, pp. 148-170.

Sweet D.J. and Bastien R.B. (1991) Use of an ABS plastic ring as a matrix in the recovery of bite mark evidence. *Journal of Forensic Sciences* **36**: 1565–1571.

Sweet D.J. and Bowers C.M. (1998) Accuracy of bite mark overlays: a comparison of five common methods to produce exemplars from a suspect's dentition. *Journal of Forensic Sciences* **43**: 362-367.

Sweet D.J. and Hildebrand D.P. (1999) Saliva from cheese bite yields DNA profile of burglar. *International Journal of Legal Medicine* **112**: 201-203.

Sweet D.J. and LeRoy H.A. (1993) Human bite marks - Victim evidence recognition and recovery. *Royal Canadian Mounted Police Gazette* **55**: 4–7.

Sweet D.J. and LeRoy H.A. (1996) Human bite marks - Recovery of forensic evidence from suspects. *RCMP Gazette* **58**: 2-7.

Sweet D.J. and Shutler G.G. (1999) Analysis of salivary DNA evidence from a bite mark on a submerged body. *Journal of Forensic Sciences* **44**: 1069-1072.

Sweet D.J., Lorente J.A., Lorente M., Valenzuela A., Villanueva E. (1996) Forensic identification using DNA recovered from saliva on human skin. *Advances in Forensic Haemogenetics* **6**: 325-327.

Sweet D.J., Lorente J.A., Lorente M., Valenzuela A., Villanueva E. (1997) An improved method to recover saliva from human skin: the double swab technique. *Journal of Forensic Sciences* **42**: 320-322.

Sweet D.J., Lorente J.A., Lorente M., Valenzuela A., Villanueva E. (1997) PCR–based typing of DNA from saliva recovered from human skin. *Journal of Forensic Sciences* **42**: 447-451.

Sweet D.J., Lorente M., Lorente J.A., Valenzuela A., Alvarez J.C. (1997) Increasing DNA extraction yield from saliva stains with a modified chelex method. *Forensic Science International* **83**: 167-177.

Sweet D.J., Parhar M., Wood R.E. (1998) Computer-based production of bite mark overlays. *Journal of Forensic Sciences* **43**: 1046–1051.

Webb D.A., Pretty I.A., Sweet D.J. (2000) Psychological aspects of bite marks and biting behaviours: a call-to-arms from forensic investigators. *Journal of Aggression and Violent Behaviour* (*Submitted*).

Wolff D., Kennedy R., Lounsbury E., MacMaster G., Olthuis K., Sweet D.J., Tutt A., Yamashita B. (1998) Dental casting materials for the recovery of tool mark impressions. *Royal Canadian Mounted Police Forensic Identification Research and Review Section Bulletin* **43**.

Wong J.K., Blenkinsop B., Sweet D.J., Wood R.E. (1999) A comparison of bite mark injuries between fatal wolf and domestic dog attacks. *Journal of Forensic Odonto-Stomatology* **17**: 10-15.

DNA profiling in forensics

J.J. Cassiman

Katholieke Universiteit Leuven - Belgium
Faculty of Medicine
Centre for Human Genetics

There is little doubt that the use of DNA analysis in the identification of individuals involved in crimes or misdemeanours, as a proof of biological paternity, in the study of population genetics and human diversity, and in the analysis of remnants found at archaeological sites has become an important tool which has added a new dimension to the methods available up to now. While the structure of DNA has been known for over 40 years we had to await for the advent of appropriate molecular methods and for the correct information about the sequence of some DNA fragments before DNA analysis could be applied to the above mentioned topics. Moreover what can be said for human DNA will in many cases be valid also for animal, plant and insect DNA as well as for the study of microbiological organisms.

DNA and inheritance

When a sperm fertilizes an egg, the fertilized egg, which is the beginning of a new life, will contain 50% of its genetic information, which it received from the mother through the egg, and 50% of its genetic information, which it received from the father through the sperm. This genetic information is contained in the DNA, which is composed of two times 3.10^9 nucleotides or base pairs. This DNA is divided in 46 fragments, which at cell division will become visible as chromosomes. In this nuclear DNA a female embryo will carry 2 X chromosomes while a male embryo will carry an X and a Y chromosome. In addition to the nuclear DNA the fertilized egg will carry hundreds of mitochondria that contain a series of small ring-like structured DNA molecules. These mitochondria are exclusively delivered to the fertilized egg by the oocytes and are therefore exclusively of maternal origin. The fertilized egg will then start dividing, leading to the formation of all tissues and organs of the embryo, the fetus and the newborn. Before each division, the DNA will be carefully duplicated. The sister chromatids of each chromosome will carry this DNA to each daughter cell after they are released from each other by the split of the chromosome centromere during the anaphase of the mitosis. As a result, all the cells of the newborn and of the later adult will thus carry the same DNA as the fertilized egg. This means that any cell of the body at any time of the embryonic development or of post-natal life can be used to determine the composition of the DNA of an individual. Depending on the circumstances and the availability of particular tissues in forensic cases one can either use blood, saliva, sperm cells, bone and even teeth, to determine the composition of the DNA of an individual. Since saliva is easily obtained from living individuals, this biological fluid is used preferentially to study the DNA. In cases however, where only skeletal remains are available, the bones and the pulp of the teeth can be used successfully to perform a DNA analysis. To make the DNA available from these biological specimens all contaminating nuclear and cytoplasmic proteins have to be removed, followed by the specific amplification of particular DNA fragments, which will reveal a unique profile of the individual.

Polymorphic fragments in the DNA

The human genome project aims at identifying the full sequence of the $3x10^9$ base pairs of human DNA and will identify many differences which exist between individuals, in their DNA composition. This project is still racing along and will reach its first completion some time in 2000. In the mean time however, it has become clear that different regions of the DNA are composed of fragments which vary in composition and in length. It was A. Jeffreys who in 1984 showed that a whole family of those polymorphic fragments could be visualized in one assay. By hybridising a single probe to a DNA preparation, a large series of DNA fragments could be visualized. Each set of fragments was typical for an individual. This 'genetic fingerprint' method has now been almost completely replaced by the use of another method, which will amplify simultaneously a series of different DNA fragments. These fragments are also composed of a series of different nucleotides that form units that repeat themselves a number of times. These fragments will therefore have lengths that vary from individual to individual. The first generation of these fragments, the variable number of tandem repeats (VNTR), were composed of fairly large repeating units of 1 0 to 20 or more nucleotides resulting in a variable length of these fragments after amplification. When a series of these fragments were amplified a unique profile for each individual could be obtained, providing that a sufficient large number of fragments were analyzed. These fragments can be visualized after gel electrophoresis on classical agarose or polyacrylamide gels or on sequencing gels. The VNTR have now been almost completely replaced by short tandem repeats (STR) which are composed of 3 to 4 nucleotide units which repeat themselves a variable number of times in the DNA of an individual. Again the analysis of a series of STR's allows one to establish a profile providing more than 1 0 to 15 of these STR's are analyzed. In addition to the STR's one can also examine repetitive sequences in the DNA that can be found at multiple places in the DNA such as the ALU sequences. Furthermore, when biological samples of males are examined, one can look specifically at a series of STR's present on the Y-chromosome. When most of the nuclear DNA is degraded, however, which is the case after death when most soft tissues have been degraded, there is still a high probability of finding mitochondrial DNA in bones or teeth. The mitochondrial DNA, which we receive only from our mother, has two regions of about 400 base pairs which form the origin or D-loop and which show a fairly high variability in their composition i.e. the sequence of the nucleotides. Analysis of this mitochondrial DNA requires amplification of this particular region and sequencing to visualise the variation in the nucleotides. As a result of the Human genome project thousands single nucleotide polymorphisms will be identified in the DNA. It is very likely that in the future combinations of hundreds of these single nucleotide polymorphisms or SNP's will be used to identify individuals or biological samples using microarrays.

Application of the DNA technology in identification

The ability to establish a genetic or DNA profile of an individual allows one to compare this profile to those obtained on biological samples presumed to be from the same individual or to biological samples of individuals who are related biologically to the individual under investigation. As a result DNA analysis can be used in paternity cases where the DNA profile of the child is compared to that of the presumed father and mother. Proof of paternity will be found when half of the DNA profile of the child is found in the mother and the other half in the DNA of the father. Maternity can be established by looking only at the sequence of the mitochondrial DNA. Here one should be aware of the fact that all maternal relatives will have the same mitochondrial DNA. So distinctions between brothers and sisters, between mother, maternal uncles and aunts can not be made based on mitochondrial DNA alone. In paternity cases where the child is a boy, the comparison of the Y chromosome DNA of the child with that of the presumed father might give additional proof of paternity. Again, since the Y-chromosome is identical in brothers, fathers and grandfathers, the Y-chromosome alone does not allow to distinguish male siblings from paternally related males. The mitochondrial DNA is also particularly useful in the analysis of hairs that every individual loses at every moment of the day. It is not surprising therefore that hairs are frequently found at the site of the crime. These shed hairs however, will usually not carry a bulb. Since the bulbar cells contain the nuclear DNA and the hair shaft does not contain nuclear DNA but only mitochondrial DNA, the analysis of these hairs usually will require analysis of the mitochondrial DNA. DNA can be extremely well preserved when kept at 40°C or when frozen at -20°C or -80°C. In biological samples excellent preservation for many years has been found in samples that dried on the air, in contrast to moist samples that are usually overgrown with bacteria and molds destroying all remaining human DNA. Since we receive 50% of our DNA from our father and 50% from our mother, we can carry only 2 variants of the same DNA fragment in our biological samples. When samples of two individuals are mixed or when DNA from one individual contaminates the sample from another individual it is not unusual to find at least three different forms of the same DNA fragment in the extract. The presence therefore of more than 2 fragments is proof for the presence of DNA of two different individuals. This is important in cases of rape, where the vaginal fluid will contain both the DNA from the victim and the DNA from the rapist transmitted through the prostatic fluid or the spermatozoa. Comparison of these profiles found with those of the suspected donors (e.g. victim and rapist) allows in most cases to conclude with high probability whether the profiles are derived from these individuals or from unidentified persons.

Contamination

As mentioned above the presence of more than 2 variants of the same DNA fragment indicates the presence of mixtures of DNA of 2 individuals or more. This contamination of the original biological specimen can occur at the scene of the crime where DNA of the victim and DNA of the perpetrator can be mixed in a single sample. However, contamination can also occur when members of the police force or of the forensic laboratories manipulate the samples carelessly contaminating them either with saliva or sweat. Finally, contamination can also occur in the laboratory when extreme care is not taken by those who handle the samples not to contaminate them. Contamination with small amounts of DNA however, is no major problem when the original sample contains large amounts of DNA since the profiles will reflect this difference in quantity of starting material. Older bone samples or even tooth samples will almost always carry some contaminating DNA on their surface. In these case the laboratory will have to take extreme care to clean the surface of these samples before extracting the original DNA. When the yield of original DNA is extremely small, even traces of contaminating DNA can interfere with a correct and authentic result. Therefore repeated analysis of the same sample and preferably of different samples from the same skeleton will be necessary as well as the quantitation of the DNA present in the sample before the result can be accepted as final and authentic.

Interpretation

DNA profiling allows one to match a biological sample to an individual as well as to exclude an individual as the donor of a particular Sammie. The success rate of these investigations will depend on the quality of the biological samples, their mode of preservation and the expertise of the laboratory. Nevertheless the results of DNA profiling should be interpreted in the context of a judicial dossier. Indeed, DNA results can confirm suspicions of the judicial authorities, can point them in a different direction from the one they were following or can make some conclusions very unlikely. Nevertheless the DNA results should not be overinterpreted and in particular should not be taken as absolute. Indeed, the value of the results depends essentially on the quality of the samples submitted for analysis. When the origin of the samples is not clear or when there are indications that the samples have been tampered with, then the DNA results may mislead the investigators. During the O.J. Simpson trial the DNA evidence was rejected by the jury although the DNA analysis had been extremely well executed. Indeed, it was argued that the origin of the samples could not be proven and that some of them had even been tampered with.

Conclusion

In conclusion, DNA analysis provides a new and powerful method to complement the existing forensic investigation techniques. While they are spectacular due their high sensitivity and high reliability they are only part of a series of investigations which should lead, when combined, to finding the correct answers to particular forensic questions.

References

Jeffreys A.J., Wilson V., Blanchetot A., Weller P., Geurts van Kessel A., Spurr N., Solomon E., Goodfellow P. (1984) The human myoglobin gene: a third dispersed globin locus in the human genome. *Nucleic Acids Research* **12**: 3235-3243.

Dental DNA evidence

D. Sweet

UNIVERSITY OF BRITISCH COLUMBIA - CANADA
BUREAU OF LEGAL DENTISTRY (BOLD)

Introduction

Tooth enamel is the hardest substance in the human body. So it is not surprising that teeth and dental structures often survive many post mortem events that can cause destruction of other tissues. Incineration, mutilation, decomposition, etc. may all subject the body to changes that make identification of the deceased person difficult or impossible. But in any case in which ante mortem dental records can be recovered, comparison of dental data can usually overcome these obstacles. Indeed, personal identification by means of the teeth is one of the most reliable methods of human identification and, as such, is the cornerstone of forensic odontology practice in most jurisdictions.

Today dentists are witnessing a significant reduction in the type and amount of dental treatment that is present in the mouths of young people. Often, children grow to adulthood without experiencing dental restorations of any kind. This fact, coupled with the fact that in some cases the destruction of the dentition by trauma or fire leaves so few dental data available for comparison to ante mortem dental records, alternative methods of identification are required. This has caused many investigators to focus on the teeth as a valuable source of DNA evidence. In fact, DNA from teeth can be used for other important reasons in addition to personal identification, such as comparison of the DNA from a decedent to biological evidence such as bloodstains, tissue samples, etc. found at the scene of a crime to link the victim to the crime.

It is important for forensic odontologists to understand the potential uses of dental DNA evidence so that when they are faced with unusual or challenging cases, possible methods to solve unanswered questions may be elucidated.

Forensic molecular biology

It is believed that the main source of DNA from teeth comes from cellular material that is present in the pulp system (nerve and blood tissue) or other cells that are trapped within the calcified tissues during dental development (odontoblasts). If these cells can be liberated, or exposed so that chemical buffers can release the DNA into solution, it will be possible using modern PCR-based analysis methods to analyse the genotype of the individual from which the tooth originates. Forensically significant concentrations of both genomic (nuclear) DNA and mitochondrial DNA (mtDNA) have been found in human teeth.

Analysis of genomic DNA using the polymerase chain reaction is the most widely used forensic test. Some controversy still exists with respect to mtDNA, especially regarding its mutation rate and degree of heteroplasmy. Thus, the following discussion will focus on the recovery and analysis of genomic DNA evidence from teeth. Furthermore, the analysis method referred to as Short Tandem Repeat (STR) multiplecing will be the focus of our attention due to its relative robusticity and specificity compared to other analysis methods.

Forensic scientists have identified many sites on the human chromosomes (loci) as being different among various individuals (polymorphic). Population geneticists have conducted studies on many human populations to determine the frequency of occurrence of these polymorphic loci in respective populations to allow statistical calculations of the relative uniqueness of a DNA profile (genotype) obtained from any one person. Most of the chosen loci are located in the non-coding region of the human chromosomes, but several are in the coding regions (i.e., vWA, FGA, Amelogenin) that produce enzymes or proteins used by the body.

Using the polymerase chain reaction (PCR), these loci can be tagged with fluorescent dyes to allow easy detection. The tagged complex can be amplified using a thermal cycler to reproduce many copies of the specific loci of interest (molecular Xeroxing). Thus, very tiny traces of genomic DNA, such as 1.0

nanogram or less, can be tested. The target DNA used in the procedure can even be partially degraded and still produce an adequate result.

DNA extraction

Initially, DNA must be extracted from the dental tissues. Dr. Sweet has adapted a technique called cryogenic grinding that uses liquid nitrogen (-186°C) to produce a brittle sample that can be pulverised in an enclosed, sterile chamber. This eliminates the possibility of contamination of the sample by extraneous DNA and also the contamination of the laboratory environment by DNA from the sample. The increase in surface area that results after pulverising a tooth or bone specimen exposes the embedded cells. An extraction buffer with a low pH can then be added to lyse the cell and nuclear membranes and liberate the genomic DNA into solution.

Using several washes and microconcentration it is possible to purify the DNA from the sample. Then the amount of human DNA can be calculated by using a human-specific DNA probe to hybridise to the DNA molecules. A light-producing reaction exposes sensitive film revealing the quantity of DNA present when compared to reference standards of known DNA concentration. Using this method, the ideal amount of target DNA can be added to the PCR reaction.

Results

The results of the PCR-based procedure are visualized using electrophoresis. This is a well-established biochemical technique that allows the fragments of DNA that are produced at the loci of interest to be separated according to size/weight and visualized so that the relative degree of rarity of the individual genotype can be calculated. One example of the electrophoresis procedure utilises a tiny capillary filled with polymer (capillary electrophoresis) as a sieve through which the various fragments can be isolated and identified. The various loci are tagged with different colours of fluorescent dyes to track the final products. Computers are used to collect the data and begin the interpretation.

It is necessary to determine the length of the DNA molecule at each forensically-significant locus following the PCR reaction because it is these data that are used to identify various individuals that may be involved in the circumstances of the case (identify a deceased victim, identify the person from which a DNA sample left at the crime scene has originated). Each cell contains information that the individual has inherited from the mother and the father at the time of conception. Occasionally, the specific information that is received at a particular locus from each parent is the same. That is, the length of the DNA fragment at that locus is the same from each parent. This is called a homozygous locus. Alternatively, each parent may contribute different lengths of DNA so that the child has two different lengths of short tandem repeating units (alleles). This is called a heterozygous locus. The frequencies of occurrence of each allele that is identified at each locus and at many different loci are used to calculate the overall frequency (rarity or commonality) of the genotype of the individual in the general population Table 1).

Table 1 – Example of a calculation of the frequency of occurrence of a genotype using the Product Rule. The frequency of occurrence of individual alleles are multiplied together to produce a frequency of occurrence for the result at that locus (p1p1 or p12 for homozygotes and 2p1p2 for heterozygotes). The frequency of occurrence of individual loci are then multiplied together to produce a combined genotype frequency.

STR Locus	Allele No. 1 (frequency)	Allele No. 2 (frequency)	Genotype (frequency)
D3S1358	17 (0.1616)	17 (0.1616)	0.0261
vWA	17 (0.2774)	19 (0.0884)	0.0491
FGA	22.2 (0.0150)	24 (0.1463)	0.0044
D8S1179	13 (0.3354)	14 (0.1890)	0.1268
D21S11	28 (0.1555)	31 (0.0945)	0.0294
D18S51	15 (0.1799)	16 (0.1829)	0.0658
D5S818	12 (0.3628)	12 (0.3628)	0.1316
D13S317	9 (0.0915)	10 (0.0457)	0.0084
D7S820	9 (0.1311)	12 (0.1280)	0.0336
	Combined Genotype Frequency =		5.1×10^{14}
	Likelihood Ratio =		1 in 19 trillion

References

Eeles R.A. and Stamps A.C. (1993) Polymerase chain reaction: the technique and its applications. Landes Company, Austin, USA.

Inman K. and Rudin N. (1997) An introduction to forensic DNA analysis. CRC Press, Boca Raton, USA.

Kirby L.T. (1990) DNA fingerprinting: an introduction. Stockton Press, New York, USA.

National Research Council (1996) Evaluation of forensic DNA evidence. National Academy Press, Washington D.C., USA.

Robertson J., Ross A.M., Burgoyne L.A. (1990) DNA in forensic science: theory, techniques and applications. Ellis Harwood Limited, Chichester.

Smith B.C., Holland M.M., Sweet D.J., DiZinno J.A. (1995) DNA and the forensic odontologist. In: Manual of Forensic Odontology - Chapter 10: DNA and forensic odontology. Bowers C.M. and Bell G.L., eds.. American Society of Forensic Odontology, Colorado Springs, USA, pp. 283–299.

Sweet D.J. and DiZinno J.A. (1996) Personal identification through dental evidence. *Tooth fragments to DNA. Journal of the California Dental Association* **24**: 35–42.

Sweet D.J. and Hildebrand D.P. (1998) Recovery of DNA from human teeth by cryogenic grinding. *Journal of Forensic Sciences* **43**: 1199–1202.

Sweet D.J. and Hildebrand D.P. (1999) Identification of a skeleton using DNA from teeth and a pap smear. *Journal of Forensic Sciences* **44**: 630–633.

Sweet D.J. and Hildebrand D.P. (1999) Saliva from cheese bite yields DNA profile of burglar. *International Journal of Legal Medicine* **112**: 201–203.

Sweet D.J. and Shutler G.G. (1999) Analysis of salivary DNA evidence from a bite mark on a submerged body. *Journal of Forensic Sciences* **44**: 1069-1072.

Sweet D.J. and Sweet C.H.W. (1995) DNA analysis of dental pulp to link incinerated remains of homicide victim to crime scene. *Journal of Forensic Sciences* **40**: 310–314.

Sweet D.J., Lorente J.A., Lorente M., Valenzuela A., Villanueva E. (1996) Forensic identification using DNA recovered from saliva on human skin. *Advances in Forensic Haemogenetics* **6**: 325-327.

Sweet D.J., Lorente J.A., Lorente M., Valenzuela A., Villanueva E. (1997) An improved method to recover saliva from human skin: the double swab technique. *Journal of Forensic Sciences* **42**: 320-322.

Sweet D.J., Lorente J.A., Lorente M., Valenzuela A., Villanueva E. (1997) PCR–based typing of DNA from saliva recovered from human skin. *Journal of Forensic Sciences* **42**: 447-451.

Sweet D.J., Lorente M., Lorente J.A., Valenzuela A., Alvarez J.C. (1997) Increasing DNA extraction yield from saliva stains with a modified chelex method. *Forensic Science International* **83**: 167-177.

Evidential value of bite marks

I.R. Hill

UNIVERSITY OF LONDON KING'S COLLEGE OF LONDON - UNITED KINGDOM
GUY'S, KING'S AND ST THOMAS' SCHOOL OF MEDICINE
DEPARTMENT OF FORENSIC MEDICINE

Introduction

Bite mark analysis has been a cornerstone of forensic odontological practice for many years. As such, it has become an established process that has proved successful in many criminal cases. However, it is not resistant to challenge and there have been many controversies (Harvey, 1976). To no small degree the arguments which have taken place have their basis in the real difficulties involved in attempting to interpret bite marks, and the often-unrealistic demands of investigators. Not infrequently in forensic investigations the police and lawyers fail to accept that the biological sciences cannot, in the present state of knowledge, be expected to deliver the exactitude of the mathematical sciences. Moreover, in bite mark analysis, the difficulties are compounded by the nature of the weapon, the characteristics of the object that is bitten and the process of biting.

This paper looks at the problems that are generated when a bite mark has to be analysed, by looking at the underlying principles. In doing so it expresses an element of caution in how bite marks analysis is reported.

Bite marks and their causation

Much has been written on this topic, both in forensic and physiological literature and so the principles are well known, thus they do not deserve repetition. There is though, one aspect of this moiety of the topic that must be considered.

There are two broad groups of bite marks, those produced in an assault and those caused during other activities, such as sexual acts and eating. Admittedly the division is not wholly distinct, because in English law no one can give consent to an act which gives rise to an injury, thus it is theoretically possible that the lawyers might argue that a love bite in which there were teeth marks constituted an assault. Be that as it may, the constructions which lawyers may place upon an act are outwitting our concerns, at least at this stage, save for one point. They illustrate the problems that exist in the study of bite marks.

The reasoning behind this division of bite marks rests in the way that the bite is caused. In an assault there is likely to be a flux of movements. The victim will be unwilling, the assailant may be in a highly excited state, as a consequence the bite mark produced will represent a contact or contacts, during a continuum of actions. Someone who bites into an apple or a piece of chocolate, for example, will probably be more considered in their actions. The greyer area occurs in consensual sexual activity, where the characteristic arousal may be expected to affect the process of biting and may involve an element of sucking. For the most part though, this activity will not mirror that seen in an assault where the participants may be more vigorous in their actions and the bite may be inflicted in a much shorter time frame. The result of this, from the forensic odontologist's point of view is that in an assault, the bite mark may be less distinct than it is in other circumstances. Definitive comparison may therefore be lacking in detail.

Analysing bite marks

The classical techniques for examining bite marks are based upon the interpreting of photographic evidence, in which a bite is compared and contrasted with the models of the teeth of suspects. One such method in which tracings of the teeth are matched against photographs of the injury has been widely used. Recognition of the potential for inaccuracy has spawned a number of alternatives, amongst which is computer analysis. The overabundance of analytical techniques available is testimony to their inadequacies, the principles of which are discussed below.

Discussion

A superficial examination of the foregoing might conclude that there is no evidential problem in bite mark analysis. Indeed with the plethora of techniques that are available to the forensic odontologist, coupled with continuing effects at refinement, there is apparently no problem. Moreover, the 'high level of scientific reliability' of bite mark analysis has made it a widely accepted adjunct to the legal process. Consequently 'the contribution that a well-executed bite mark investigation can make to the legal process is no longer questioned' (Ligthelm and van Niekerk, 1994)

Sadly, this is not the case. As mentioned briefly above, the fact that there are so many different techniques for analysing bite marks means that there is no universally accepted standard. It is certainly true to say that in many instances the commonly used method of analysis is the well-established photographic method, in which the teeth of the suspect are compared, albeit with some variations depending upon the circumstances and the particular likes of the individual expert.

If bite mark analysis is compared with haemoglobin estimation, for example, where there are standard techniques, internal quality controls and external validation of performance, it can be seen that bite mark studies are wanting. That is of course not to suggest that haematological and biochemical tests in medicine are not subject to an element of variation. They are after all measurements of biological factors. Nevertheless, they do offer a greater degree of precision than we can expect from a bite mark. This is not a criticism of the methodology or of the technical expertise of the forensic odontologist. It is merely a function of the material that they have to use.

Nambiar et al. (1995) almost achieved an explanation of the problems involved or perhaps an aspect of them. They said that 'unfortunately, in practice bite marks can never be taken to represent with absolute accuracy the dentition of the originator, particularly if it has no unusual characteristics'. This is, perhaps, a misstatement of the issue, for they were discussing not so much the representation of the bite, but more its recognition, and the two are quite different. What the authors were looking for, as all forensic odontologists do, is a way of saying that a mark undeniably comes from suspect A and not suspect B. In so doing they are saying that no one else could possibly have made that mark.

Bite marks manifest considerable variation in their appearances, depending upon a wide range of factors such as the area bitten, the way that the biting was done, the force used and the health of the victim. All of which take no account of the perpetrator's dentition. Nor do they allow for any change in shape of the bite mark, which may occur from changes in position, thus a round bite mark may become oval. This can occur if, for example, there is a round mark on the upper arm. Extension of the arm stretches the skin and the mark becomes oval. Circumstantial and anatomical variability, combined with pathophysiological changes contrive to present the forensic odontologist with an unenviable task. A task, which belies the apparent complacency manifest in the praise, heaped upon the bite mark analysis.

Part of the problem lies in the court's demands for absolutes in an area wherein precision may be an unattainable ideal. It is to some extent a characteristic of the way in which forensic science has developed. In recent years DNA and other analyses have given a degree of certainty which could not have been hoped for in the past and this has reflected upon other disciplines. However, all is not as it seems. The probability of a chance DNA match in one case was said to be 20 million to one. As a critic of this statistic said, the fact that the defendant and two other people in the United Kingdom could have committed the offence is not as impressive (Watkins, 2000). Placed against this, what then can be said of bite mark analysis, in which an often diffusely bruised area or a curved surface on a body undergoing post mortem change?

Clearly the forensic odontologist has to be given the greatest help. If he cannot attend the mortuary, then good quality photographs must be taken. These should not distort the mark and there should be a scale attached. If at all possible the area should not be dissected. Removing the skin releases the tensions in the tissues and causes the wound to alter shape, added to which, any shrinkage in the skin due to post mortem change will alter the shape and dimensions of the wound. Moreover, if the bite is on a curved surface, flattening out would dramatically alter the appearances. In such a situation, the experimental accuracy demonstrated by Whittaker (1975) in which two examinees subjectively matched 98,8% of wax impressions to study models would surely be unattainable. If this level of accuracy is regarded as a bench mark, then that would seriously negate other, less accurate diagnoses. Whittaker showed the fact that purely visual matching is much less accurate in the same study where he found a 30% fall in right answers.

Clearly what this shows and what has been argued many times, is that a range of factors have to be considered (Whittaker, 1975). These have been mentioned above, but Levine (1977) added a new area, the position of the body when the bite was inflicted. This is always going to be difficult because in an altercation there may be a wide range of movements between those involved. As these are likely to be taking place in an atmosphere of heightened tension, followed by mixed emotions, memories are likely to be poorly formed. Even if all of the variables can be taken into account and measurements such as arch curvature, tooth width, angulation and spacing are used there is still an element of art in the science (Levine, 1977; McGivney and Barstey, 1999). Implicit in this is the criticism in the problem of reproducibility and storage of information, which makes comparative studies difficult. It has been suggested that digital imaging removes subjectivity (Naru and Dykes, 1996), others have stated that computerised mathematical techniques may be helpful (McGivney and Barstey, 1999).

Conclusions

It can be seen that far from being the easy concept that some authors would seem to state, bite mark analysis is complicated by a range of variables. These are compounded by the diversity of analytical techniques available to the forensic odontologist, and despite mathematical modelling and computerisation the picture is not showing signs of real improvement. This is not a unique position. A recent survey of opinions on shoe marks showed that different observers came to different conclusions (Shor and Weisner, 1999). Forensic odontologists have made strenuous efforts to improve the reliability of bite mark evaluation. Courtroom successes have imbued the topic with a degree of accuracy that, if it were achievable, would arguably be almost as enviable as DNA analysis. This is clearly not the case. It is extraordinarily difficult to achieve consummate accuracy in the biological field, for there are too many variables. An indistinct mark, ambiguous individual characteristics in a particular mark, the possibility of change of shape and a host of other factors all mean that some caution must be expressed. There is no room for complacency in bite mark analysis.

References

Harvey W. (1976) Dental Identification and Forensic Odontology. Henry Kimpton Publishers, London, United Kingdom, p. 120.

Levine L.J. (1977) Bite mark evidence. In: Symposium on forensic dentistry: legal considerations and methods of identification for the practitioner. Standish S.M. and Stimson P.G., eds. *Dental Clinics of North America* **21**: 145-158.

Ligthelm A.J. and van Niekerk P.J. (1994) Comparative review of bite mark cases from Pretoria, South Africa. *International Journal of Forensic Odonto-Stomatology* **12**: 23-29.

McGivney J. and Barstey R. (1999) A method for mathematical documenting bite marks. *Journal of Forensic Sciences* **44**: 185-186.

Nambiar P., Bridges T.E., Brown K.A. (1995) Quantative forensic evaluation of bite marks with the aid of a shape analysis computer programme. Part I. *International Journal of Forensic Odonto-Stomatology* **13**: 18-25.

Naru A.S. and Dykes E. (1996) The use of digital imaging technique to aid bite mark analysis. *Science and Justice* **36**: 47-50.

Shor Y. and Weisner S. (1999) A survey on the conclusions drawn on the same footwear marks obtained in actual cases by several experts throughout the world. *Journal of Forensic Sciences* **44**: 380-387.

Watkins S.J. (2000) Conviction by mathematical error. *British Medical Journal* **320**: 2-3.

Whittaker D.K. (1975) Some laboratory studies on the accuracy of bite mark comparisons. *International Dental Journal* **25**: 166-171.

The balance of DNA and bite marks
A Lawyer's point of view

M. Bowers

Forensic science has numerous specialities that sometimes overlap. Footprints, tool marks and fingerprints have casually been considered analogous to bite mark analysis by some authors. I do not adopt this simplistic view. Since my tenure as a Diplomat of the American Board of Odontology, I have never seen a bite mark case that equals the rigor of Known sample comparisons normally performed in these other fields. Quite often the odontologist in the United States simply uses a single set of dental casts taken from a suspect developed by law enforcement. We now have bite mark cases that have potential DNA results. Is there something lacking in odontology? I certainly think so. This overlap is here to stay and every odontologist needs to consider its ramifications.

Footprint analysis uses dental materials. Fingerprint analysis uses areas of similarity or concurrent 'points' to quantify the degree of 'match' between Known and Questioned evidence samples. Odontology in the United States and Canada tried this approach in the late 1980's with bite mark scoring guidelines. Inter-examiner consistency was found to be lacking and the idea was quickly dropped. Analysis of fibres and ballistics use the optical comparison microscope. Some dentists use wax Xeroxing and hand tracing while others use computers to do comparisons digitally. The modes of analysis for the physical comparison 'sciences' are boundless. Completing this array of forensic overlaps is biological evidence. Bite marks are having a honeymoon relationship with DNA identification. This article discusses this particular overlap. I also have a few suggestions about the use of computers rather than wax exemplars and mechanical measuring tools.

A dilemma or just business as usual?

When DNA results are pending what is the optimum protocol when an odontologist is retained to compare a suspect (hopefully hidden in a large representative sample) to a definite bite mark? The purists would say the two fields of physical matching and DNA analysis are independent. The literature suggests that the investigation of a bite mark be independent of extraneous information to prevent either intentional or expectational bias. Knowing a suspect was caught crawling through the window doesn't add weight to an otherwise nonprobative bite mark in skin or an inanimate object.

The legal consumer of expert testimony and opinion expects odontological testing to be independent and blind to other expert conclusions. This is despite the fact that physical matching of bite marks is a non-science, was developed with little testing, and has no published error rate. Anecdotalism and a minuscule number of inadequate population studies support our efforts. The purveyors outweigh the sceptics, however, and the field still marches on. In a nutshell, what is the frequency of occurrence for a rotated left maxillary central incisor present in adult males who have diastemata? Beats me. Subgroupings of racial differences? I don't have a clue. Someone who has a bit of financing for such things will have these delving for future investigation.

Alternatively, DNA has arrived on the criminalistics scene and in relatively short order well-established guidelines and laboratory safeguards are in print. The statistical justification for DNA identification has been scrutinised and approved (with attending argument) through rigorous testing and technique standardisation. Variegated racial groups possess population frequencies for their polymorphic loci that have forensic significance. Is this field an able ally or a forensic competitor? I do believe it is a little of both.

What then, should a prudent odontologist do in this situation? The temptation to create an opinion early in an investigation is normal. Who wants to say that odontology cannot conclusively establish a bite mark as unique? We are trained to accomplish this if the evidence is 'good'. It is left to the individual dentist to determine what is sufficient evidence for this determination. This is the foundation where a fragmentary or unclear bite mark develops into a 'positive or probable match' between common dental characteristics.

The greater experience of one expert over another has been argued as a guarantee of a 'better' result. This is unproved conjecture and serves as the single support for proponents of the non-science approach. The interpretation of a bite mark case must be determined by methods that are reproducible and obvious. The 'I can see it, you can't?' school of expertise will not lead us into the 21st century. Instead, it will spell the doom of this particular aspect of crime investigation.

An opinion is worth nothing unless the supportive data is clearly describable and can be demonstrated in court. How does one weigh the importance of a single rotated tooth in a bite mark when the suspect has a similar tooth? The value judgements range widely on the value of this feature. This is not science. Instead, statistical levels of confidence must be included in this process. Until then, the DNA results are far superior to the odontologist's position. There is no honest way to deny this.

You may form an opinion before the DNA results are in, but the majority of cases will be proven conclusively by the biological tests. This presumes they are performed. If the two independent tests do not correlate, I hope odontologists will not rely on the theory that there were two assailants involved in the same case-one biting and the other spitting.

The majority of bite mark casework does not have accompanying DNA evidence to provide either additional confirmatory support to the prosecution's odontological argument or exoneration of a defendant. Legal argument contesting or advocating bite mark opinions has a distinct disadvantage since the current discipline lacks quantitative methods and statistical confidence levels. The courtroom argument will consider the reliability issues on the proffered opinions as a factor of a dentist's years of experience and credentials rather than a critical review of scientific methods that have been tested validated and then duplicated in the odontologist's laboratory.

This is not the case regarding the use of the forensic application of DNA analysis to forensic casework. The decade-long use of biomolecular methods to individualise crime scene samples of blood, semen, sweat, bone, tooth fragments, dental pulp, saliva, hair, fingernail and dandruff has motivated the creation of TWGDAM. Pronounced 'twigdam', this acronym stands for Technical Working Group for DNA Analysis Methods. Major crime laboratories in the US and Canada formed this committee to reflect on the currently available DNA multiplex systems, methods, and interpretative assumptions. Their recommendations for approved methods include limits on the use of population statistics derived from the numerous comparative studies of allele frequencies found in diverse ethnic and geographical communities. Early in the 1990's, the National Research Council established a 'ceiling principle' when population studies were scant and fragmentary. This produced a conservative estimate of mathematical calculations derived from the multiplication of individual allele (gene) probabilities determined at various places (loci) in the human genome (the 23 pairs of chromosomes). For example, if allele X is found in 0.012 of the target population and allele Y shows up in 0.34 of the same population, the two values are multiplied together (the 'product rule'). This assumes the two alleles occur independently in the population (Hardy-Weinberg Principle). Odontologists do the same when two or more dental characteristics of interest are reflected in both the Questioned and Known samples. The problem is lack of knowledge regarding this linkage and the likelihood of someone else having the same collection of toothborn characteristics. Its time for a TWGDONT to be constructed. The odontology opinion is conjecture until proven otherwise.

The combination of DNA and bite mark opinions

Casework involving both forensic dentistry and molecular biology is increasing. Biological and patterned tooth mark evidence, when recovered from the same site at a crime scene or autopsy suite, will result in parallel analyses. These events create new issues regarding odontological testing protocols and examiner ethics. This section briefly reviews two instances where both forensic dentistry and molecular biology became intertwined due to the nature of evidence found at crime scenes and on a homicide victim. This duality of evidence may be derived from a common origin such as a bite mark on skin. Similarly, an inanimate object connected to the scene might possess tooth marks and biological material that will enable two investigators to be working towards independent conclusions. Law enforcement will expect reports from both sources to correlate the physical and genetic data developed from a suspect. Regardless of their point of view, the odontological investigation must be independent and shielded from DNA results until the dentist has reached a final conclusion.

The forensic literature in the later 1990's contains compelling evidence of DNA analysis being used in conjunction with conventional bite mark and human identification casework. DNA techniques are considerably more tested than bite mark analysis and have been adopted for paternity determination, biomedical research, and serological comparison of known and unknown blood samples. In light of the oft-quoted 1993 Daubert US Supreme Court decision mandating a scientific analysis of scientific expert opinion, bite mark interpretation has been scrutinised in print by few forensic practitioners and fewer United States courts in this context. Up to now, bite mark analysis has escaped the strictures applied to this decade's judicial review of DNA identification methods. The odontologist, when asked to perform a physical comparison between Questioned and Known evidence in a case containing additional DNA testing, may end up supported, or possibly in conflict, with the biomolecular results. The various commercially available multiprobe PCR systems' power for discrimination and stringent validation process may support or repudiate the odontologist's conventional physical comparison methods. A conflicting result will, at the very least, reduce the weight given to the odontologist's results. Because of this potent scientific competition, the proponent of bite mark conclusions faces an ethical challenge.

Case One

A murder victim had been bound and gagged with commercially available duct tape. Marks of five upper teeth were clearly evident on the surface of the duct tape along with the impressions of the lower front teeth showing on the inner cardboard spool apparently made by the assailant when he used his teeth to tear the tape. A forensic odontologist was retained by the prosecution to compare the pattern in the tape to a suspect's teeth. The suspect had two fractured upper front teeth, which compared favourably in size and position to the marks on the tape. Direct physical comparison and a video superimposition of the suspect's dental models were made with a duplicated model of the marks on the tape. The odontology report concluded, with a high degree of certainty, that the suspect's teeth made the indentations in the tape. Prior to the odontologist's analysis, the questioned tape had been swabbed and genomic DNA was obtained and profiled. A DNA report was submitted after the odontological result had been established. The DNA analysis confirmed the odontological findings by concluding the suspect's salivary DNA was on the duct tape. The suspect was tried and convicted of second-degree murder. The odontologist was not aware of the availability of DNA evidence until after the trial.

Case Two

A total of 23 cigarette butts were recovered from a crime scene and a vehicle as part of a homicide investigation. Small folds were noticed at the end of two filter tips that strongly suggested they were created by the edges of two teeth. The prosecution forensic odontologist opined that a certain suspect could have made the bite marks on the filters. The defense odontologist analyzed the same evidence and excluded the suspect. PCR analysis was then performed on saliva recovered from the filter material. The suspect was eliminated as the source of DNA on the filtertip.

Discussion

The odontologist faces a critical point when presented with a case that involves both the physical comparison of a questioned bite mark to known teeth and the potential of DNA results from related evidence. Nordby has outlined the outside influences that affect expert testimony and noted pre-established expectation-laden observations as one such factor. Good scientific practice avoids bias and pre-judgement of data in clinical and lab experimentation by using single or double blind strategies that attempt to obtain pure data observations and control external influences. Forensic casework is simply another form of experimentation, which requires independent analysis and independent interpretation by investigators. Examiner ethics advocate that a case requiring multiple investigations be bifurcated in order to counteract bias from crossover influence between the interpretative and analytical methods. First, the odontologist performs the systematic physical comparison of the pattern injury or mark with plaster models of known teeth. The DNA results are intentionally left unknown to the dentist. The important feature of this protocol is to keep the odontologist blind to the DNA results. This sequence of events assures the criminal justice system that the results are independent. If interexaminer contamination occurs, the expert opinions will be linked, resulting in the DNA being independent and the dental assessment being tainted. The court use of expert testimony requires that the participating scientists come to trial free of this flaw.

What do can non-biotechnic people do?

The following discussion indicates that physical comparisons may be bolstered with digital analysis that takes the odontologist to the computer rather than to the tracing board. For once maybe everyone will follow the same technique and get similar results.

Digital Analysis of Crime Scene Evidence using Adobe PhotoShop®

There are advantages to the application of Adobe 5.0 Photoshop® in the visual comparison of two and three-dimensional physical evidence obtained from forensic investigations. This material focuses on bite mark evidence but is applicable to other areas of investigation. Forensic examiners can easily master the techniques and should consider this methodology to standardise analysis procedures and to document quantitative and associative results. Step-by-step procedures performed digitally include:
-    Capture of original crime scene images digitally or through conventional photography.
-    Scanning two and three-dimensional images of bite marks.

- Scanning dental casts.
- The use of Photoshop® to adjust the acquired image contents to perform the following
- Rectifying certain types of perspective distortion.
- Resizing of the injury or crime scene photograph to any desired magnification.
- Fabrication of suspect dentition (or recovered objects) overlay exemplars for physical comparison with questioned pattern injuries on skin and other substrates
- Comparison techniques using Photoshop® that can be used to associate or exclude evidence through metric measurements and non-metric shape association.

It has been shown in 1998 that the fabrication of dentition overlays using this method produces more accurate results than other traditional means. The adaptation of additional Adobe Photoshop® features permits the odontologist to digitally continue the physical comparison process throughout the entire case. What are some of the issues involving digital imaging?

Gaining control over your images

Traditional photography has the investigator waiting to evaluate the pictures until the photo lab has processed the film. The use of video cameras has eliminated some of this waiting, but a high definition photograph is what we need in bite mark casework. A crime scene video image isn't going to be the final exemplar of a patterned injury, footprint, or mark.

The traditional adage of 'take more pictures than you need' is also used to minimise this problem. Usually one or more of a myriad of conventional film pics captures the prerequisite detail, colour balance and has the proper scale and film to object plane perspective. I would say this is not always the case and this poses the strongest advantage for adopting digitisation methods.

Original crime scene photographs come in all shapes and colours. Off-angle (or angular) distortion is a common occurrence. How many tripods have you seen in use at crime scenes and in the autopsy room? The use of circular reference targets in the two-dimensional ABFO No. 2 scale was intended to allow the photo lab to correct for this type of distortion. Going digital with a camera or a scanner allows the person responsible for the total investigation to control this variable.

If you have a digital image, you can use image-editing software like Photoshop® to eliminate a number of other photographic problems. Out of focus shots can be sharpened. Poor contrast, colour balance correction, cropping out unwanted elements, adding text, and other editing actions are better controlled.

Inclusion of images in reports and other communications

Pictures embedded in the case report allow for better communication with your clients. The transfer of image files via the Internet creates a direct connection with colleagues in a matter of minutes. It is fast and convenient and is already well established and in use by odontologists linked via the World Wide Web.

Comparison techniques via computer

I have spent many hours looking at Questioned and Known evidence samples through a comparison microscope. It is valuable, but what can you get from it? Most times a Polaroid or 35mm picture. What do you do next? Pull out the protractor and ruler to attempt measuring angles and distances directly from the picture or its magnified duplicate. You can draw lines with a Sharpie pen. Are these measurements the same between examiners? I doubt that two or more people would collect this data exactly the same in every instance.

Digital imaging permits the computer to be your comparison microscope. A high resolution scan of a suspect's teeth or a hollow volume overlay may be compared to a bite mark in skin or inanimate objects like a cigarette filter tip. Photoshop® allows both images to be properly sized and then superimposed or compared side to side. You like to work at 3x-life size? 300 % magnification is only a mouse click away.

Metric analysis is the next big advantage of digitisation. Photoshop®'s Toolbox contains features that allow both the Questioned and Known samples to be measured independently and then compared. Tooth dimension and angulation relative to the X-, Y-axes may be developed for both samples. Grids and rulers may be placed in each image. The days of the protractor, compass and Boley gauge are long gone if you want them to be.

Reproducibility and consistency between examiners

I touched on this before but I want to emphasise it as another positive aspect of digital imaging. Photoshop® records each step taken by the examiner in the application's History Palette. This file may be saved and included with the final images and conclusions. This creates a total record of what was performed and makes irrelevant the dreaded 'touch-up' or 'enhanced' argument against digital imaging. It also places multiple dental examiners on the same analytical playing field. The endless comparison techniques allowed in bite mark analysis are a major deterrent in this field's march towards consistency between dentists. These computer techniques are not 'high-tech' to the point that the average dentist cannot possess the equipment and skills necessary to produce a good product. Testing of equipment (calibration), methods (validity and reliability) and additional training are the key concepts of forensic investigation.

What are the negatives to digital imaging?

Print quality

What is easily seen on your computer monitor is not necessary what your printer will output. Manufacturers have considerably improved desktop printers in the recent past but photo quality printers are not cheap. If your equipment or budget is not up to it, an alternative is to have a professional imaging lab print the final image files for you. Print quality is not a factor when producing an overlay of teeth for printing on clear acetate. A struggle might ensue, however, when printing the image of the suspect's teeth or the Questioned pattern.

Original image quality

Images from lower-priced digital cameras will cause problems regarding close-up focusing, lens distortion and low resolution. This aspect is directly related to your budget when you are the original source of evidence photographs. Don't forget to test a lot of cameras before you buy one.

The alternative here is to keep using conventional photography and later transfer the images to digital for image analysis. This is a realistic stance adopted by certain law enforcement agencies and equipment manufactures such as Polaroid and Kodak.

Image file size

Multiple high-resolution images need huge amounts of disk storage space. This requires a digital camera with LARGE capacity when multiple images are captured. Alternatives are to take a laptop computer with you to accept uploading from the digital camera. If you don't have a laptop carry enough digital camera memory cards to reload during the collection of evidence.

Learning Curve

Becoming a digital photographer and image analyst does involve learning some new concepts and skills. But, really, I don't think many of us in odontology are resistant to getting new tools and learning how they work. It seems a common trait of our profession.

21st century techniques and DVI standards

Digital imaging: uses and potential abuses

R. Wood

PRINCESS MARGARET HOSPITAL - CANADA
DEPARTMENT OF DENTAL ONCOLOGY
DENTAL AND MAXILLOFACIAL RADIOLOGY

Photography and radiography are the result of the use of similar end-image capture systems (film or digital image capture). This is where the similarity ends. Whereas photography, digital or not, is the result of the encoding of reflected light off of a surface, radiography is a measurement of the differential penetration or absorption of an x-ray beam by an absorber, which in our case is a patient. As such, a radiographic image is essentially a partially penetrating shadow captured, usually on film, or occasionally on direct digital imaging systems.

Video capture of oral and facial photographic images is used for patient presentation, medico-legal reasons and insurance claim justification. This image capture can be taken from digital videotape or static images from an intraoral camera. Intraoral cameras are becoming a routine part of private dental practice especially in geographic locales where increased numbers of dentists practice as well as in affluent practices. Such images can be captured for electronic storage on a number of different media and viewed later or archived for long term storage. Alternately the images may be printed on photographic paper and kept in hard copy format in a patient's chart. The advantage of having a digital storage mechanism is the ability to transmit such images to distant sites for second opinions or insurance claim fulfilment (so-called tele-dentistry), preserving the image for later comparison (before and after treatment), reduction of physical storage requirements, and the ability to manipulate these images to enhance the information they contain. Most intraoral cameras have an attachment for acquiring facial photographs, intra oral photographs, as well as recording images from conventional dental radiographic views. Some systems have an integrated means of recording x-radiographic images along with photographic images in a master patient file.

Both digital dental radiographic image capture and intraoral photographic image capture are physically impressive to student, practitioner and patient alike and may one day become part of every dental office. This being said there is no real reason for either of these technologies to exist. Digital radiography is known to result in less exposure to the patient but patient doses are exceptionally low already, especially if we elect to use inferior E speed film. Dental practitioners are already using extremely low exposures for our conventional images. With the doses currently used we couldn't measure any reduction in cancer induction by lowering them further even if dentists were all to immediately switch over to digital imaging systems (Tannock & Hill, 1987; Kondo, 1993; Preece, 1997). With respect to caries diagnosis using digital systems, Wenzel (1998) noted that there was no evidence from clinical studies that the number of retaken images was reduced, no evidence that the systems are sufficiently robust for daily clinical use, and little evidence that enhancement features are used in making clinical treatment decisions.

Indirect digital dental radiographic imaging is accomplished by digitising pre-existing hard copy images by way of a desktop scanning system. Versteeg et al. (1 997) describe the advantages and disadvantages associated with direct and indirect digital radiographic imaging techniques. Chief among the disadvantages associated with indirect digital radiographic imaging was the necessity of retaining the x-ray processor and its associated chemistry. If conventional analogue images are digitised however the process may still be more economical. Commercially available scanners have been reduced in price about eight times since their introduction to where they are easily within the financial grasp of most practising dentists. So how can we use these systems in forensic odontology?

Image enhancement can be undertaken with either photographic or radiographic images. Contrast and density can be changed as well as the part of the H and D curve we wish to focus on. For example it may be advantageous to view the radiolucent (dark) parts of a radiographic image rather than the lighter ones. Digital image analysis, direct or indirect, allows us to do this. In addition we can readily magnify images for closer view and highlight portions of images for closer inspection. This may allow forensic dentists to utilise 'smiling' ante mortem facial photographs to assist in the identification of found human remains or to sanitise injuries to accident victims which allow their publication in the lay press (Perper and Backner, 1992). Examination of the palatal rugae for identification purposes as proposed by Kogan and Ling (1973), can be simplified by use of scanned images of these anatomic areas. Digital images of the palatal rugae and morphological features of the teeth may permit ante mortem and post mortem digital comparison with either measured metric evaluation or pattern analysis using subtraction techniques or side by side comparison techniques. Most commercial desktop scanners will allow scanning of three-dimensional objects with excellent three-dimensional representation of measurements. This may be checked by comparing scanned images of known dimensions at varying distances from the scanner surface.

Forensic dentists may also use digital images of dental radiographs to assess the spatial relationships of the root complexes when comparing ante mortem and post mortem images. To do this we can use subtraction techniques in which an ante mortem radiographic image is photographically inverted and then compared to a digital image of the same area by assigning 50 per cent opacity to each. If the case is a match then the combined images will cancel one another out leaving for display only those areas, which are not identical between the two images (Wenzel and Lis, 1994). Alternately we can select a horizontal section of a root complex in a radiograph of a posterior jaw and assess the degree of fit between an ante mortem and post mortem image (Tai et al., 1994). This has allowed identification of humans where there was little or no interventional dental treatment. This technique is useful in the paediatric and permanent dentitions and not useful in the mixed dentition because of the radical spatial changes seen at this stage of dental development (Wood et al., 1999). In cases where dental intervention is present along with radiographs digital dental radiography allows for the assessment of the similarity between small areas on the ante mortem and post mortem radiographs. Importantly, the use of digital radiography is not restricted to small areas of dental radiographs. It is well known that the frontal sinus region of the skull for example may possess enough inherent and differing features from one person to the next to allow person identification (Harris et al., 1987). Forensically significant extra-gnathic sites such as the paranasal sinuses can be compared where digital images are present or can be acquired by scanning pre-existing radiographs. Pattern and metric analysis of the frontal sinus region can be assisted by indirect digital dental imaging and side by side comparisons. Ante mortem images in the form of direct digital imaging, conventional film or microfiche can serve as a source of comparative material.

Computer-assisted tomography (CT scanning) is essentially a form of digital imaging in which volume portions of a patient (voxels) are converted to picture elements (pixels) each of which is assigned a CT number, which reflects the average atomic weight of the volume element. CT scanning can be used to assess the degree of fit between a hard or stable soft tissue wound and a suspected weapon. In most instances the weapon is metallic and is not amenable to CT examination because of its excessive atomic weight. The materials knowledge of the forensic dentist allows the reproduction of the exact contours of a weapon in a bony-tissue-equivalent material which, when placed in the gantry of a CT scanner and suitably scanned, allows for the assessment of whether a weapon could have produced a particular hard tissue or soft tissue injury (Wood et al., 1996).

Similarly, digital images of soft tissue injuries may also allow assessment of the conformity of a soft tissue injury to the dentition of a suspect in the case of bite mark examination or alternately the degree of conformity between a hard object which may have been impressed into soft tissue (Wood et al., 1994; Sweet et al., 1998).

The use of digital image information is not restricted to the comparison of patterns nor to metric analysis. An alternate use of scanned dental images is the assessment of colour and colour changes. Root colouration as an indicator of dental ageing was originally proposed by Ten Cate et al. (1977). At the time of this study the quantification of colour was problematic because of the arcane technology available. A reassessment of Ten Cate's collection of extracted teeth of known age was recently undertaken by the author and has been submitted for publication (Lackovic and Wood, 2000). In this study the degree of colour change in the sub-gingival root portion of extracted teeth of known age was assessed. The root surfaces of these teeth were evaluated for the degree of colour saturation (cyan, magenta, yellow, and black). In each gender and for each colour there was progressive increase in root colouration, which correlated very well with patient age. The correlation coefficients for these groups of teeth were all in excess of $r = 0.89$ and a linear model could be applied to this data. Such a model should allow the ageing of an unknown set of human remains and such a study is currently underway.

Uses of digital photography in mass disaster situations may present both opportunity and hindrance. At the Swissair 111 air crash off of Canada's east coast, digital images of forensically significant tattoos, jewellery and other personal effects were recorded and kept for comparison purposes. Such images could be 'cleaned up' in a manner making them suitable for viewing by survivors and next of kin. The use of digital cameras allowed semi-real time photographic comparison.

What then are the drawbacks or problems with digital imaging systems?

The main drawback to digital imaging systems is their lack of uniformity of image storage type. In the jurisdiction in which the author works the radiographs and images are the property of the patient and must be transferable and transportable in suitable format for use by the next treating dentist. The storage of digital data may not be transferable to another office if the equipment is not identical and will be useless if the new treating dentist uses analogue imaging systems. This portability will create major problems in mass disasters since the mass disaster information officer for incoming ante mortem information will likely not be able to accommodate the numerous digital imaging systems from around the world. Clearly we need every digital imaging system to have a single storage mechanism to allow transfer as well as a means of allowing production of high quality printed images of what they contain.

Another problem with digital imaging systems is the ability to alter images to the benefit of the immoral practitioner and to the detriment of the innocent patient. This has been done already, admittedly with indirect digital image methodology (Sinton et al., 1997; Tsang et al., 1999). The use of altered analogue images is easier to detect than the use of digital images whose programs may allow enhancement and even painting. Security measures must be improved in digital imaging systems to make the images unalterable.

One cannot prevent a determined, talented and deceitful practitioner from defrauding his victim. A problem arises however in the apparently innocent manipulation of digital images in cases where a match is attempting to be made. This may occur in cases of bite mark comparison. In the digital analysis of bite mark comparison, there are frequently manipulation and enhancement of the images done with a mind to improving the quality of the image for comparison purposes. In such cases the defence should have access to unaltered analogue images so that they can examine both the results and the methodology used by the prosecutor's expert. If the defence receives only digital images then he or she cannot be sure they have not already been manipulated. The forensic dentist must be aware that guides aiding lawyers in cross-examination of experts with respect to electronic evidence already exist (Gahtan, 1999). In the future we can expect to be examined more diligently when digital images form the basis of our opinion.

Conclusion

In summary forensic dentists require a uniformly accepted image format which is unalterable and transportable. In the absence of such a system we require photographic evidence on analogue film, a history of the steps undertaken at each stage of the comparison process and justification for the alterations made. Forensic dentists need to have a means of assessing the work-product in digital imaging or scientifically be able to reproduce similar results given the same initial data. As a group we need to have clearly-defined areas of image manipulation which are generally regarded as permissible as well as guidelines as to what is not acceptable.

References

Gahtan A.M. (1999) Electronic Evidence. Carsweil, Toronto, Canada.

Harris A.M.P., Wood R.E., Nortje C.J., Thomas C.J. (1987) The frontal sinus: forensic fingerprint? A pilot study. *Journal of Forensic Odonto-Stomatology* **5**: 9-15.

Kogan S.L. and Ling S.C. (1973) A new technique for palatal rugae comparison in forensic odontology. *Canadian Society of Forensic Sciences Journal* **84**: 3-10.

Kondo (1993) Health effects of low-level radiation. Kinki Press, Osaka, Japan, pp 143-164.

Lackovic K. and Wood R.E. (2000) Changes in root colouration as an indicator of chronologic age. (*Submitted*).

Perper J.A. and Backner J.S. (1992) Visual identification from videotape after electronic erasure of mutilating injuries. *American Journal of Forensic Medicine and Pathology* **13**: 309-314.

Preece J. (1997) Exploding the myth of diagnostic radiation risks. In: Advances in Maxillofacial imaging. Farman A.G., Ruprecht A., Gibbs S.G., Scarfe W.C., eds. Elsevier Press, Amsterdam, The Netherlands, pp 413-420.

Sinton J., Wood R.E., Pharoah M.J., Lewis D. (1997) Digital image manipulation in the diagnosis of caries on bitewing radiographs.*Oral Surgery Oral Medicine Oral Pathology* **84**: 443-448.

Sweet D., Parhar M., Wood R.E. (1998) Computer-based production of bite mark comparison overlays. *Journal of Forensic Science* **43**: 1046-1051.

Tai C.C., Blenkinsop B., Wood R.E. (1994) Computerised digital slice interposition in dental radiographic identification: Case report. *Journal of Forensic Odonto-Stomatology* **11**: 22-25.

Tannock I.F. and Hill R.P. (1987) The Basic Science of Oncology. Pergamon Press, New York, USA, pp 122.

Ten Cate A.R., Thompson G., Dickinson J., Hunter H. (1977) The estimation of age of skeletal remains from the colour of roots of teeth. *Canadian Dental Association Journal.* **2**: 83-86.

Tsang A., Sweet D., Wood R.E. (1999) Potential for fraudulent use of digital radiography. *Journal of the American Dental Association* **130**: 1325-1329.

Versteeg C.H., Sanderink G.C.H., van der Stelt P.F. (1997) Efficacy of digital intra-oral radiography in clinic dentistry. *Journal of Dentistry,* **25**: 215-224.

Wenzel A.A. and Lis A. (1994) A quantitative analysis of subtraction image based on bite wing radiographs for simulated victim identification in forensic dentistry. *Journal of Forensic Odonto-Stomatology* **12**:1-5.

Wenzel A. (1998) Digital radiography and caries diagnosis. *DentoMaxilloFacial Radiology* **27**: 3-11.

Wood R.E., Miller P.A., Blenkinsop B. (1994) The use of image editing techniques for computer assisted bite mark analysis in a case of self defence biting. *Journal of Forensic Odonto-Stomatology* **12**: 30-36.

Wood R.E., Chiasson D., Blenkinsop B., Brooks, S.E. (1996) Use of computer- assisted tomography in wound weapon matching in cases of fatal skull injuries. *Canadian Society of Forensic Science Journal* **29**: 49-55.

Wood R.E., Kirk N., Sweet D.J. (1999) Digital dental radiographic identification in the pediatric, mixed and permanent dentition. *Journal of Forensic Sciences* **44**: 910-916.

Teledentistry in Disaster Victim Identification (DVI)

S. Kortelainen* and E. De Valck

KEMI - FINLAND
HEALTH SERVICES

In Disaster Victim Identification (DVI) the latest telecommunication equipment offers a lot of opportunities to increase the quality and improve the efficiency of the Disaster Victim Identification Team's work. In this presentation we describe the past and present of telemedicine, the high-tech in dentistry today, and the use of telematic equipment in disaster victim identification work.

Telemedicine has been reality for some 15 years, but the cost of the prototype hardware and software has been prohibitive for individual doctors. In addition to the cost, the learning curves were daunting to many of professionals. A lot changed in the last three years. With the advent of interactive office computer system, voice-activated programs, comprehensive databases, and various other technological goodies, electronics have become a critical part of today's successful practice. The newest communication technology offers facilities for quick health data transmission. It is necessary though to improve the confidentiality and user-friendliness of these applications and systems which should provide easy access to health data in real-time. In particular, real-time translation capability is required in emergency cases, where quick access to the existing health data and the possibility of teleconsultation improve the quality of diagnoses and the accuracy of treatments.

Telemedicine is examination, treatment and follow-up of the patient, as well as training both patients and personnel by using telematic systems, which enables an easy access to expert opinion regardless the location of the patient (Van Goor and Christensen, 1992). In a simple way it means to move the data, not the patient. Already in 1924 on the front page of Radio News there was a vision of a radio-doctor, who could be in connection with his patients via voice and image. The first TV transmissions where done three years later in 1927. However, the technology was not yet ready to get the visions to reality until a couple of decades later. In the 1950's telemedicine was started in the United States with radiographs, which were transmitted via radiowaves. In the 1960' s and 70's telemedicine was applied in Canada and Australia, which are huge countries, and thereby benefit a lot from telemedicine. In Europe the most active countries have been France, Norway and Sweden. However, from the Scandinavian countries, Finland was the first to test telemedicine back in 1969. The real big bang in telemedicine has occurred in the 1990's due to the vast enhancement of the teletechnology.

There are lots of applications for telemedicine. Videoconferencing is a very suitable way of consulting a specialist, getting a second opinion, having meetings at different places at the same time, advising the patient or teaching the personnel. Videoconference-technique is also used in telepsychiatry. Teleradiology is another very widely used application. Digitised x-rays can easily be transmitted. The amount of digitised radiographic equipment has increased rapidly during the last years. Also digitised still pictures and videoimages and microscope slides can be transmitted to get an expert opinion. The emergency units are able to transmit biosignals, like EEG or ECG, to the hospital, and get advises from the doctor. Dental data, electronic patient files, digitised x-rays, intra- and extraoral images, are suitable to be filed and transmitted with the modern teletechnology.

Telemedicine has many advantages. The most important benefit is the improved quality and effectiveness of treatment. The patient gets the right diagnosis and treatment fast, and if needed, getting an expert opinion or a second opinion is not dependent on the resources of the clinic. That enables better equality to citizens, also to those living in remote places. However, there are some facts, which slow down the expansion of telemedicine. The investments are high at the beginning, but in a long run the expenses per unit are lower than in traditional medicine. It would be essential to have integrated standards. There exists the variety of equipment, applications, and software, which might not be compatible. Joint international standards, like DICOM and HL7, would guarantee a much better situation for the users instead of the law of the jungle. Confidentiality, data security is highly important, when dealing with delicate health information. As long as we are acting in Intranet, there should be no big problems, but in an Internet environment, many questions have to be solved concerning trustworthiness. As our personal abilities and attitudes to use modern teletechnology differ, time is needed to train the professionals to efficient use of these systems. The trend towards user-friendly applications and equipment is very welcome.

In dentistry the high-tech tools have become more and more common use. Electronic patient record-keeping programmes, digital radiography, and suitable software help the doctor in his/her diagnosis and treatment planning process. The new technology offers effective tools for demonstrating the value of dentistry to the patient, for building a better doctor-patient relationship, for creating a demand for professional treatments, and services offered by the practice. Intraoral cameras, interactive multimedia patient education systems, and cosmetic imaging software enable to visualise the patient's mouth condition and make them better understand. In the U.S. almost half of all general practitioners are using an intraoral video system in their practices. Also the use of digital radiography is increasing by a few percentage per year (Dental Products Report, June 1999). Europe is following the trends rapidly. In the near future the special demand for wireless applications will increase, because of the mobility of people and availability of suitable technology. The GSM network covers all the urban and most rural areas of Europe, and the network coverage is expanded continuously. New techniques will be introduced to enhance the data transfer rate more than ten-fold, which improves the suitability of technology for medical data transfer.

For many people the world has become their village in the last decades. Increasing travel for business or holiday purposes have become everyday life in our part of the world. Subsequently the increase in car, train, boat and aeroplane traffic has of course resulted in a greater number of major disasters where there have been people from different nationalities among the victims. One of the major problems that the Disaster Victim Identification Teams in the different countries have been dealing with, is the availability of personal, medical and dental data. In all these cases there is mostly a great pressure from the family members and everybody involved in all the handling processes of such disasters is under scrutiny of the media. That is why it is of major importance from a legal and human point of view that the victims can be positively identified as quickly as possible. The key to this identification is very often the access to and the transmission of ante mortem data of the victims. As these data are of course very personal and confidential there is a great need for a system that can cope with the legal requirements regarding this matter.

The development of teletechnology, and the increased use of it in the dental clinics enable the use of those techniques also in DVI-work. The present methods of getting ante mortem data via telefax, mail or personal delivery are useful, but the modern teletechnology makes the procedure many times faster, reliable and efficient. The original data will never get lost, because they will stay filed in the clinic. The wireless applications make impossible to register the post mortem data straight to the computers on the field. The digitised images of the bodies and digitised x-rays of the teeth can easily be filed into the laptops together with the other obtained information. The problems rise in the variety of the equipment, systems and the software used in the disaster victim identification. At the 11th Meeting of the Standing Committee on Disaster Victim Identification in Lyon, 1999, was decided to recommend, that a system of transmission of information for DVI be approved that is: a) accessible, b) linked to the Interpol Intranet 'ATLAS' system, c) linked to the DVI 'IDDONT' system, d) linked to the 'telnet' system, e) compatible with all of the above. TelDent is a model of transferring dental and medical data in a confidential way for the comparison phase of Identification.

Great attention has to be paid to the confidentiality of transferring delicate health information. In the DVI-work the legal and ethical aspects of each country involved have to be respected. In the countries of the European Union the protection of privacy and personal data has to follow the national legislation and Directive 95/46/EC of the European Parliament and the Council (24 October, 1995) on the protection of individuals with regard to the processing and the free movement of personal data, and Directive 97/66/EC of the European Parliament and the Council (15 December, 1997) concerning the processing of personal data and the protection of privacy in a telecommunication sector. European Commission has dedicated millions of Euros for projects promoting user-friendly information society, and especially to innovations on trustworthiness and reliability.

TRANSMISSION OF DATA
in Disaster Victim Identification

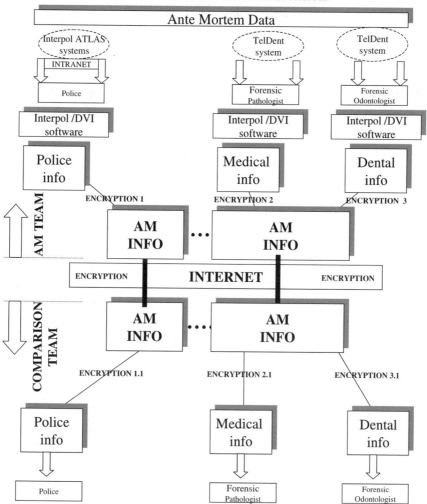

Fig.1
Transmission of data in Disaster Victim Identification

Conclusion

In conclusion, the vast enhancement of high-tech applications, software and equipment used in dentistry enables lots of new possibilities to improve the quality of Disaster Victim Identification work. To maximise the benefit of those, there exists a need of new investments, unified standards, and training of the users.

References

Van Goor J.N. and Christensen J.P. (1992) Advances in medical informatics: results of the AIM exploratory action. IOS Press, Amsterdam, The Netherlands.

DVI interpol procedures. The police

J. De Winne

NATIONAL POLICE FORCES - BELGIUM
COMMANDER OF THE DISASTER VICTIM IDENTIFICATION TEAM - BELGIUM
PRESIDENT INTERPOL DVI STANDING COMMITTEE

Introduction

The Belgian Disaster Victim Identification Team was founded after the disaster at Los Alfaques in 1978.

At that time Interpol put together a commission, which purpose was to standardise the international forms on which personal information of the people involved in mass disasters had to be filled in: the ante mortem and post mortem forms.

This commission also created a manual for practical use: Manual on Disaster Victim Identification, which was internationally distributed in November 1986.

The Belgian DVI-Team was put into action for the first time in ZEEBRUGGE when the Ferry 'Herald of free Enterprise' capsized on March 6th 1987. In this disaster, 189 bodies were recovered and positively identified.

Consequently, conclusions were drawn, and the initial organisation of the DVI-Team was modified.

Up to December 31st, 1999 the team has been put in action on 116 occasions. In total 463 victims were identified by the Belgian DVI Team. We had to deal with a variety of disasters, as well in size as in the nature of the disaster. An explosion in a shooting club in Brussels, a hotel fire in Antwerp, an explosion and fire in the restaurant of a truckstop in Eynatten, an aeroplane crash in Bucharest (Romania), several big traffic accidents with heavily injured and burned victims. The team was also put into action on request of the International Criminal Tribunal for the former Yugoslavia (ICTY), for the search, gathering of evidence and the identification of murder victims, buried by the perpetrators in massgraves in Kosovo.

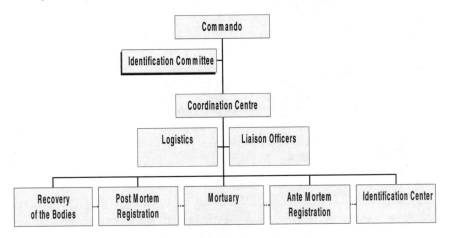

Organisation of the DVI team

This organisation consists of a commando to which is added: A co-ordination centre, responsible for all administrative and logistic tasks. Liaison-officers, taking care of contacts with foreign police forces and other organisations that are involved in the handling of the disaster. There are also five work-units: the Recovery Team, the Post Mortem Team, the Ante Mortem Team, the Identification Centre, the Reception Team.

Tasks

The different units each have their specific tasks.

- The Recovery Team

  The main task of this team is the recovery of victims at the disaster site. Several teams search the area, after having gritted the disaster area into a number of numbered sectors. Each recovered body or body part is numbered, photographed and removed from the recovery area to a gathering point and transported to the Technical Identification Zone.

- The Post Mortem Team

  This team is active in the technical ID zone. Each body is described, externally and internally in co-operation with pathologists and odontologists. All information is transmitted onto the Interpol post mortem forms. Samples for DNA - analysis are taken. Specific characteristics are photographed. Fingerprints are taken. The clothes are also described and afterwards cleaned, so that they can be returned to the relatives after identification. The jewellery and other valuable objects are registered and photographed. After a last check the post mortem-forms are taken to the Identification Centre, and put into a specific computerprogram.

- The Ante Mortem Team

  In the mean time our liaison officers at the information centre of The Social Intervention Services of the Belgian Red Cross have tried to establish a list of the probable victims of the disaster. This ante mortem information is gathered in co-operation with the Social Intervention services of the Belgian red Cross, who are in contact with the relatives of the victims. This service is staffed by people with an education as social workers and psychologists, who have received special training in this kind of matters. The ante mortem forms are put into a central computer, just like the post mortem forms.

- The Identification Centre

  The identification is done at two levels: First of all, some fifty parameters that feature on the ante mortem and post mortem forms are automatically compared with each other by a specially designed computer software. This results in a probability score concerning the identity of the unknown bodies. The identification itself is done by a careful manual comparison of the information on the ante mortem and post mortem forms by the different specialist groups involved in the identification and the individual results are debated by the ID-Committee. This committee consists of: The DVI Commander, the chief pathologist, the chief odontologist and the head of the ID centre. When there is the slightest doubt about the identity, the data are reviewed and if any doubt remains about a 100% positive identification, comparison of DNA material will be applied. The results of this comparison are sent to the judicial and administrative authorities that have to draft the death certificate.

- The Reception Team.

Their tasks are divided in three parts and are executed in co-operation with the Social Intervention Service of the Belgian Red Cross. First off all they will question the members of the family who came to the disaster area, in order to collect as much ante mortem information as possible of the presumed deceased victims. They also secure the mortuary area, where the bodies are taken, after they have left the technical Identification Zone. On request, after positive identification, a visual contact with the deceased, by the relatives is possible. This will be done in the presence of a member of the Reception Team.

How is the DVI-Team put into action?

When a disaster occurs in Belgium, the local police of the disaster area can ask for assistance from the DVI-Team. At that moment the DVI organisation is put in alert. This means they have to be able to get to the disaster area and start working within six hours after the alert.

When a disaster, involving Belgians, occurs abroad, the plan Simonet can be put into action. The Ministry of Foreign Affairs can subsequently decide to send a polyvalent team to the disaster scene. This may consist of members of the Department of Health, the Red Cross, Civilian Defence, and the commander of the DVI-Team. The Belgian Air Force provides transport and logistic backup. The most important task of this polyvalent team is to collect as much information as possible, in co-operation with the local authorities. The Belgian authorities will then be informed whether further assistance needs to be sent to the disaster area. In the mean time, the DVI-Team is kept on stand-by and ready for departure to the disaster area.

Collaboration with other services

Such a difficult and stressing task cannot just be accomplished by the DVI-Team alone. A good collaboration with other services and organisations is absolutely indispensable. In this spirit we have the co-operation of pathologists, forensic
odontologists and forensic anthropologists. Civilian Defence takes care of the transport of bodies from the disaster area via Technical Identification, to the

mortuary. They also provide the DVI-Team with special equipment, and take care of the catering.

The Belgian Red Cross can also be called in for help: The helpservices take care of the transport of the bodies within the technical Identification Zone. The Social Intervention Service is responsible for the information centre. It offers its co-operation for gathering ante mortem information and communication with the victims' relatives.

The Armed Forces can also be called in for logistic support and specialised personnel.

Remarks

The identification of the victims of a disaster is not really very difficult to organise, but the practical execution is rather very complex.

The key problem in the whole identification process is to gather correct ante mortem information. So it is necessary to have a pre-organised plan and well-trained personnel, who pay attention to every little ante mortem and post mortem detail or element that can help to identify a body. Flexibility and co-operation as a team with the other specialists involved in disaster management on an interdisciplinary base are the factors to success.

The main philosophy of the whole process has to be that we are serving the relatives of the victims and that everything has to be done for their relief.

A special concern has to be taken in the psychological assistance of the team members, because the work is very stressful. During the operation each head of a working unit is also responsible for the well being of his team members.

There is also a real need to give people the opportunity to express their emotions. Therefore it is absolutely necessary to organise a post-operational psychological debriefing, apart from the operational debriefing.

DVI interpol procedures. The medical examiner

W. Van de Voorde

KATHOLIEKE UNIVERSITEIT LEUVEN - BELGIUM
FACULTY OF MEDICINE
CENTRE OF FORENSIC MEDICINE

Introduction

In case of a mass disaster the judicial authorities (prosecutor, judge of investigation) will appoint the 'experts' needed to investigate the cause of the disaster and to identify the victims. Mostly, the Disaster Victim Identification section of the federal police and one or more physicians, preferably forensic pathologists, will be ordered to investigate the case. Once nominated, the forensic pathologist will function as the medical examiner.

Necessity of identification

Identifying every single victim is a major and exigent task for the authorities. Determining the identity of a person is necessary for:
-   psychological reasons

The process of mourning only can start when one is convinced that his or her relative is one of the victims. They need to know! Therefore, everything has to be done to give the relatives the opportunity to take leave of the deceased.

- administrative purposes
  A death certificate is needed to bury a relative. Certifying death and giving the authorisation for burial is the task of the registrar. He therefore needs an official declaration of death (form 'model III C or III D) filled in by the treating or examining physician. Without identity the death can not be registrated and no regular authorisation for interment or cremation can be given. The medical examiner has the duty to fill in the official form used to declare a certain person to be dead, and consequently bears the responsibility in Death Certification.
- judicial reasons
  Legal authorities will investigate for the cause at the disaster, wanting to know if prosecution of responsible(s) is warranted. In case of prosecution, it is important to know the number and identity of the victims of the 'criminal offence'.

The role of the medical examiner

The role of the medical examiner is double. He/she has to examine the cause and manner of death, i.e. an aircraft crash may be caused by a heart attack of the pilot, and has to identify officially the victims, necessitating the assistance of other investigators (DVI, odontologist…). In optimal conditions, the medical examiner co-ordinates, together with the DVI, all investigations concerning the corpses.

Methods to identify human remains

In mass disaster, bodies mostly are heavily injured, mutilated, fragmented and spread over a large area. Personal belongings (jewellery, clothes, eyeglasses…) may be damaged and disrupted from the body. Besides premortem injury and post mortem mutilation, examination may be hampered by burning and charring.

The medical examiner/forensic pathologist has to examine the scene where he/she can be most helpful in recognising and recovering human remains. He/she may assist at the numbering of the corpses; the scene will be mapped and photographed (overview and details) by the forensic photographer (DVI). It is of utmost importance that each 'number' (corresponding to a specific recovering) can be related to a specific place on the map: personal objects, body-fragments…

are most likely to be found in the vicinity of the corresponding corpse (trunk). A thorough and detailed search of the spot where a specimen is found is necessary in order to look for the smallest object such as teeth, keys... All recovered and numbered human remains are to be stored at low temperature (± 5 °C) and transported in sealed bags to a well-equipped mortuary, if necessary 'build' at the spot.

The forensic pathologist will proceed in detailed medical examination, including full autopsy performed on every corpse. The pathological examination will be documented with photographs, at least colour facial photo (if appropriate) and personal characteristics (jewellery, scars, tattoos…).

The medical examination includes
- complete, detailed inspection of the body to gain a general description (height and weight, race and gender, age, hair colour and length, colour of eyes, moustache and/or beard, perforated earlobes…), to recover every peace of clothing and personal objects and to look for specific characteristics such as scars, tattoos, piercings, prostheses…;
- complete autopsy to determine cause / manner of death (investigating the pattern of injury) and to search for previous surgical procedures (sterilisation, osteosynthesis devices, mechanic prosthetic valve, vascular prostheses, breast amputation, pacemaker…), pathologic anatomical findings (diseases?); inspection of the internal genital organs may be necessary to determine gender;
- scientific identification methods:
  - fingerprints (dactyloscopy): assisting in obtaining fingerprints if possible
  - odontology: assisting the forensic odontologist by preserving upper and lower jaws, eventually completed with radiology, for odontologic comparison, ageing of the individual and DNA-fingerprints
  - genetics: obtaining blood or tissue (even teeth and bone) for DNA-fingerprints, also from undetermined/unrecognisable human body fragments
  - eventually special techniques
  - radiology: for comparison with ante mortem radiographs, especially cranium (sinus frontalis and dentition), and determination of age (and sometimes gender)
  - anthropology: examination of bones may give information about race (cranium), gender (cranium, pelvis), age and height (length of long bones such as humerus and femur)
  - computer-assisted image analysis (superimposition, facial reconstruction).

Identification is essentially based on comparison of ante mortem and post mortem data. The more points of concordance and the rarer a particular finding, the higher the probability that (the remains of) a victim can be identified. General profiles based on description of found bodies may help in selecting possible candidates for identification by ante- and post mortem comparison from a list of missing persons. Scientific certitude of a certain identity may be obtained by dactyloscopy, forensic odontology and DNA study. In a lot of cases a high probability is gained by the forensic pathologist when a (nearly) perfect match is found; in all instances his/her post mortem findings are at least needed in selecting the missing persons whose ante mortem data have to be compared. As much important, of course, is to get detailed ante mortem data which mostly is the task of authorities (police, i.e. DVI).

A disaster most likely is a non-announced and overwhelming event, so procedures are necessary. For the purpose of identification in such difficult circumstances, the Disaster Victim Identification team has developed a procedure based on the Interpol guidelines for identification of disaster victims. Two detailed (separated) forms will be used to gather and notify all necessary ante mortem and post mortem data, to be completed by police officers, forensic odontologists and forensic pathologists (medical examiners). After a sufficient matching is obtained, a 'certificate of identification' is signed by the responsible police officer, pathologist and odontologist. It is important that besides obtaining as much detailed data as possible, one realises that also the comparison of the data is teamwork and has to be completed by all responsibles, chaired around the same table. According to Belgian law, once a 'certificate of identification' is obtained in case of a disaster victim, the medical examiner can sign out the declaration of death form that allows death certification and burial authorisation by the registrar (after approval by the prosecutor).

Conclusion

To benefit the best results concerning the identification of disaster victims, a multidisciplinary approach is needed, based on expert knowledge and co-operation between all members of the identification team. This physically and psychologically demanding task asks from every member the capacity to work in a spirit of understanding and equality, in a well-organised disciplinary context along the guidelines as stated in the manual of Interpol and as applied by the Disaster Victim Identification section of the Belgian federal police. The process of identification; ideally, starts with an expert investigation of the scene, followed by gathering as much detailed ante and post mortem data as possible, completed by a multidisciplinary comparison in search of as much matching data as possible, and all this in the shortest time possible.

DVI Interpol procedures. The forensic odontologist

F. Prieels

Introduction

Disaster Victim Identification, normally the responsibility of the Police, is a difficult and demanding operation that can only be brought to a successful conclusion if properly planned which of necessity has to involve the active participation of many other agencies. It is, however, only one aspect of dealing with disasters which will all vary considerably in extend and effect, but the identification procedures can always be utilised irrespective of the number of victims involved.

The ultimate aim of all DVI operations must invariably be to establish the identity of every victim by the comparison and matching of accurate ante mortem and post mortem data. The three major phases involved in victim identification are: procurement of ante mortem information for possible victims (ante mortem information); recovery and examination of bodies to establish reliable post mortem evidence from the deceased (post mortem information); and comparison of ante mortem and post mortem data to positive identification of each body.

In order to achieve, maintain and improve standards and facilitate international liaison, Interpol recommends the formation in each member country of one or more DVI Commissions. They should have a responsibility not only for disaster response, but also for the vital functions of pre-planning and training of key personnel who may, by virtue of their position, suddenly become involved in, or responsible for one or more of the many aspects of the disaster, including DVI. The identification procedures assume an organised intervention; they are intended to serve as a sound basis upon which to develop DVI practices. The advice may be of particular help to those member countries not having a permanent Disaster Victim Identification Commission.

Documentation

The Interpol Standing Committee on DVI has developed and refined internationally agreed Victim Identification Forms that, in practice, are equally applicable in cases involving single unidentified bodies and multiple fatalities. Use of these forms by all member countries will not only ensure that comprehensive information is obtained, but will greatly facilitate the transmission of identification data between member countries. It is on the basis of these forms that ante mortem and post mortem data recording is done. The Interpol Victim Identification Form consists of several sections – divided in two groups: yellow forms for listing latest known data concerning a missing person, and pink forms for listing all findings concerning a dead body. The F1 and F2 section of the AM and PM forms should be recorded by the forensic odontologist and contain dental information or dental findings. The layout of the AM and PM Forms is the same, to facilitate comparison. The standard of dental data varies not only between different dentists, but also between different countries; for that reason the two digit FDI system is used in the Interpol Forms. In forensic identification it is justifiable to use professional abbreviations for the description of dental findings, provided they leave no doubt about their correct interpretation. A list of abbreviations with explanation is then necessary. Unfortunately there is no worldwide list of abbreviations in forensic identification and no standard list exists in Interpol.

Identification methods

Accurate identification is achieved by matching ante mortem and post mortem data obtained through circumstantial evidence (e.g. Personal effects such as clothing, jewellery and pocket contents.) and physical evidence from external examination (e.g. fingerprints), and internal examination (e.g. medical evidence, dental evidence and laboratory findings.)

Dental evidence is a particularly important and effective method of identification. The examination of teeth and jaws can only be properly carried out by a forensic dental expert. Because of the exact detail which can be obtained from this examination it is accepted procedure for dental experts, when necessary, to remove teeth for sectioning and age evaluation, or jaws (complete or in part) for maceration and radiography. On site x-ray equipment will be of great advantage in dental examination. It is recommended that x-ray equipment, preferably portable, is always made available in the mortuary. Additionally, genetic identification techniques provide a powerful tool for diagnostics in legal medicine that can successfully be applied to the identification of disaster victims.

Genetic identification techniques currently in use complement other methods commonly used for disaster victim identification, especially when the body has been severely mutilated. Obtaining, storing and analysing these samples, from both the victim and potential relative, requires special expertise and should always be undertaken by a scientific or medical expert.

Victim identification

Missing persons branch

A missing persons branch will be devised into an ante mortem Record Section and an ante mortem File Section. The primary function of this branch will be to establish, as soon as possible, a reliable victim list. When specific medical and dental information is required, it is important to obtain names and addresses of family doctors and dentists (present and past), together with the best possible medical and dental history. This is done by the ante mortem Records Section. The ante mortem File Section will file all ante mortem reports alphabetically under name. This section is responsible for checking that all ante mortem records are complete and for obtaining any missing data. An ante mortem Medical Unit and an ante mortem Dental Unit should be set up, consisting of qualified doctors and dentists entitled not only to read the records, but also capable of interpreting and extracting relevant information. These expert groups will need to cooperate closely with the corresponding post mortem Medical and post mortem Dental personnel. Both expert groups should be responsible for filling in the respective parts of the DVI post mortem form.

Victim recovery

It is essential for search teams to understand that they are the first of many links in the identification process, and that the accuracy with which they undertake their commitments may mean the difference between success and failure. Medical personnel may accompany them.

Mortuary branch

The post mortem Records Section is responsible for collecting the post mortem descriptions and findings for each individual body. In case of a mass disaster, it can be expected that dental examination may delay the flow of bodies through the examination room. If required, the post mortem Dental Unit will arrange for dental X-ray apparatus to be set up in a convenient place within the examination room. It will be responsible for X-ray film processing and adding any additional information to the descriptive section of the DVI post mortem Form. Finally, if teeth or jaws are taken out of the body, the unit will again be responsible for all further handling and for additional data being properly recorded.

Identification centre

This centre compares ante mortem and post mortem documents, forwarded from the ante mortem and post mortem File Sections. The Identification Centre can save considerable time by using a computerised matching programme able to quickly suggest the most likely possible matches and establish potential eliminations with a high degree of probability. It is essential to remember that any computer programme is an aid and that final conclusions and decisions can only be made by the forensic experts. In the ID Dental Section, a large number of exact details can be compared. The amount of work involved will dictate the number of specialists who will be required. A possible procedure to be used in the comparison process is to display on a AM record and the team of dentists to then compare the PM records that they have completed. This will also give them the opportunity to discuss and agree their findings.

Comparison of reports

The two reports (AM and PM) can easily be compared as the general set up is the same. For mass disasters it has been suggested to use characteristic details for rapid sorting. Concordant details can be extracted from the reports. These should be used in the evaluation of the probability of the identity. Details are often divided into ordinary and extraordinary type. Details occurring less frequently than in 1/10 of the population may be considered extraordinary. The comparison should result in a conclusion of the odontologic evidence. There are 4 different grades on our conclusions as recommended by Interpol.

The odontologic identity is established when we have more than 12 uncharacteristic concordant features or a probability of <1/10000 that another person might fit these features. In these cases we may conclude that the possibility of mistake is so small that we can exclude it. The odontologic identity is probable if there are between 6 and 12 uncharacteristic concordant details or the probability of a wrong identification is estimated to be <1/100. In these cases the odontologic evidence is strong but needs support by other evidence such as physical features or technical findings to establish the final identification. The odontologic identity is possible when we have 6 or less concordant details or the probability of making a wrong identification of >1/100. Finally, the identity can be excluded. In fact, these are the only cases where we can give an absolute sure conclusion on a scientific base.

Conclusion

The role of the forensic odontologist in identifications is quite important: in recording ante mortem and post mortem data, as well as in comparing those data. A good collaboration between the different DVI experts is necessary to obtain a good result.

References

Guide to disaster victim identification. Interpol 1996.

DMORT- The U.S. model for mass fatality incidents

J. Kenney

DMORT - USA
FORENSIC ODONTOLOGIST

Beginning in early 1990, the National Funeral Director's Association (U.S.) funded the beginnings of a portable morgue for use is mass fatality incidents. Only mortuary supplies and services were provided, no forensic expertise or supplies were included in the assembled kit. Prior to that time, at each mass fatality incident that occurred, rapid assembly of the necessary components of a temporal morgue occurred. Depending on the locale, resourcefulness of the local coroner/medical examiner, their disaster preplanning and training, the facility and equipment available would vary widely. The only continuity in these activities resulted if the airline that was involved had recently experienced an accident, the same funeral services company was engaged, or consultants in forensic identification (odontology in particular) were hired by the affected airline. Usually disaster management fell to the airline's medical director and safety office. While some individual airlines had safety/disaster manuals available

they were only a few pages thick, and did not address the post mortem operation
at all. The outside consultants hired by the airline often worked in concert with a
local coroner or medical examiner's staff, consultants or volunteers to direct the
operation and provide counsel to the medical examiner or coroner who found
himself with anywhere from dozens to hundreds of fatalities literally dropped into
his jurisdiction. Today, as a result of the U.S. Family Assistance Act of 1996, all
commercial airline companies based in the U.S. or foreign flag carriers flying into
the US must have a comprehensive disaster plan in place. These family assistance
activities fall under the purview of the National Transportation Safety Board.

As an example, in 1979 in Chicago, a complete temporary morgue was
established at an American Airlines Hangar at O'Hare. Due to the fact that it was
a major maintenance and operations base for the airline, all of the building trades
were available to run electrical wiring, plumbing, and construct light stanchions
or what ever else was needed to begin the necessary identification work. Medical
x-rays were taken in the company medical department on the second floor of the
hangar. A Phillips Dental X-ray and Peri-pro processor unit were donated by a
local dental supplier. Ironically and sadly his daughter perished on the flight.
Banquet tables were used as autopsy tables, and an entire side of the hangar, large
enough to hold 2 DC-10's side by side was utilised from 25 May 1979 through 15
July, 1979 when the operation was moved downtown to the medical examiner's
office. This was according to the medical examiner, 'the largest temporary morgue
in history'. An odontologist with extensive experience in disaster identification
and morgue management was hired by the airline to advise and assist with the
operation. A funeral service company also was hired by the airline's insurance
underwriters to handle disposition of the remains of the 273 victims. Both worked
in close concert with the local chief medical examiner, and his staff and chief
odontologist. The FBI Disaster Squad provided fingerprint expertise, and later in
the investigation, a forensic anthropologist and radiologist were added to the
scientists present in the morgue.

In 1995, American Eagle lost an aircraft with 72 on board. It plunged into
an Indiana newly harvested soybean field on Halloween. The local coroner, a
dentist, did not normally see 72 deaths in a full year in his county. Resources were
offered to the coroner, but until the FBI Identification Team arrived, everything
was on hold. The only major decision that had been made was to use the local
high school field house as the temporary morgue. The field house was directly
attached to the school, and the cafeteria was in the next room. The coroner stated
'The FBI has arrived and they will handle everything'. This was a nice thought,
but untrue, as the FBI mission was to provide fingerprint identification capability,
not manage the operation for the coroner. It also took a lengthy argument with the
coroner and county sheriff to convince them that there would be identifications
made from the shattered remains of the plane and its victims, and that it was
crucial to grid or stake the crash site. The staking of remains led to the locating of
three dental fragments that allowed three more victims to be identified and

returned to their loved ones. The location of the morgue was also discussed with the coroner and sheriff and then changed to a military reserve training facility about 30 minutes south of the crash site and well away from the high school. The NFMC portable morgue was dispatched to this location and used very successfully.

In September of 1990 a Memorandum of Understanding (MOU) was signed between the National Funeral Director's Association and the National Disaster Medical System (NDMS) a branch of the US Public Health Service. The NFDA split off a separate foundation, the National Foundation for Mortuary Care in the early 90's to directly supervise, equip and deploy the morgue. It was stored at Sky Harbor Airport in Phoenix, Arizona. As a result, a new MOU was signed with NFMC and DMORT in 1993 and continued until 1998. The first deployment was the Hardin Missouri Cemetery Flood Disaster. The same type of disaster occurred in Albany, Georgia the following year and again the morgue was deployed to support the DMORT Function.

Beginning with the deployment of the NFMC morgue for the US AIR 737 crash in Pittsburgh, the generosity and ingenuity of the local and state funeral director's associations caused additional major equipment to be donated or purchased for the morgue. During the American Eagle ATR 72 Indiana accident in 1994, roll-around portable autopsy tables were donated by the Indiana Funeral Director's Association. In addition, American Eagle purchased and donated the dental x-ray processor to the morgue.

The first test 'in extremis' of the DMORT came with the bombing of the Murrah Federal Building, Oklahoma City in 1995. DMORT Personnel and equipment were deployed to assist the Oklahoma State Medical Examiner. The following year saw a commuter plane ground collision with a private propjet in Quincy IL. Elements of DMORT were deployed as well as the portable morgue. In 1997 an Embraer prop-jet commuter plane iced up while executing an approach to Detroit Metro Airport and fell from the sky in Monroe Michigan. The morgue and DMORT were deployed to assist the local medical examiner with the recovery and identification of the dead scattered on frozen ground under snow that was 12-18 inches deep. In mid-summer of that same year, Korean Air 801 suffered a controlled flight into terrain at Agana Guam, and DMORT personnel and the morgue were deployed half way around the world.

The collision of an AMTRAK train and Semi-tractor-trailer 50 miles south of Chicago again brought out the DMORT Team, and the portable morgue. This was a fairly rapid operation with only 11 dead. Due to lack of hard information about passengers aboard the train, it was originally felt that there could have been dozens who perished.

The Federal Government had in the aftermath of TWA 800 and the inception of the Family Assistance Act of 1996 funded and equipped a new morgue, incorporating elements that had been refined by the NFMC's experience. Another MOU was signed between the Public Health Service DMORT and the

National Transportation Safety Board in 1997 to automatically deploy DMORT for aircraft accidents. In 1998 the sponsorship of DMORT transferred to the National Association for Search and Rescue.

In the event of a mass disaster, the various agencies of the US Government each have specific responsibilities to assume. The 1988 document that defines these roles is the Federal Response Plan. There are broadly defined areas of response, termed Emergency Support Functions (ESF's). ESF #8 covers health and medical response, which includes victim identification and mortuary services. The primary agency for ESF #8 is the Department of Health and Human Services -- US Public Health Service. Within the Public Health Service, the Office of the Assistant Secretary of Health, Office of Emergency Preparedness- National Disaster Medical System. NDMS is tasked with providing these services. The Disaster Mortuary Operational Response Team (DMORT) was developed specifically to handle the victim identification and morgue services.

DMORT is tasked to provide:
- Management of victim identification and mortuary services
- Assistance in search and recovery
- Mobile morgue
- Victim identification expertise
- Family assistance centre organisation and operation
- Ante mortem data collection
- Support personnel for DMORT team members

DMORT teams are set up on a regional basis, following the ten Federal administrative regions of the US. Team members include forensic pathologists, forensic odontologists, forensic anthropologists, fingerprint specialists, medico-legal investigators, funeral directors/embalmers and morticians, medical records specialists, radiology technicians, mental health specialists, security and administrative personnel, computer specialists, and other support personnel. Each of these team members with the exception of the MSU (Management Support Unit) is a private citizen with particular area(s) of expertise as enumerated above. They are activated and become a temporary Federal Employee. Their licensure and certification within their discipline and home state is kept current. During activation, the licensure and certification becomes federalised and valid in whatever state the person is assigned during their deployment.

The DMORT team members work in concert with local authorities to assist the coroner or medical examiner who maintains the final authority to make identifications, release remains and direct the morgue operations.

The first federally forensically assisted disaster occurred in Virginia in 1940 when a plane crashed carrying a FBI agent and stenographer. The Director of the FBI, J. Edgar Hoover became impatient at the time it was taking to return the bodies of the FBI employees back to Washington. He dispatched several fingerprint experts with copies of the employees print cards to make a scientific identification. Thus was born the FBI Disaster Squad. Because of their recurring presence at aircraft disasters, they de-facto became the 'experts' at overall management of disasters.

Military pathologists and dentists were also often called upon by local jurisdictions to assist when a disaster struck. Since many military dentists had dealt with war deceased through the Graves and Registration offices, and the Army's Identification Lab in Vietnam, or experience with high impact aircraft crashes and the resultant identification problems, they became a primary resource for trained dental identification specialists. Beginning in the mid 1960's the Armed Forces Institute of Pathology offered a formal course in Forensic Dentistry. The course included some of the first comprehensive information on disaster management. Fingerprint experts from the FBI and trained forensic dentists, especially those, who had worked several disasters, became some of the first forensic disaster managers. A forensic anthropologist who was employed by the Federal Aviation Administration at their Civil Aeromedical Institute on Oklahoma City, Dr. Clyde Collins Snow became an early expert at mass fatality identification. He participated in his first investigation in 1961. His skills would be honed to a fine point in 1979 when he spent 5 weeks working on the American Airlines DC10 crash at O'Hare.

The funeral service profession through the National Funeral Director's Association became interested in the problem as a whole in the 1980's and set up a committee on Mass Disasters. A number of individual state funeral director's associations had set up their own disaster teams. Through the pioneering work of Mr. Tom Shepardson, a funeral director from Syracuse NY, the New York State Funeral Directors Association established one of the most comprehensive mortuary disaster squads, with several truckloads of equipment. Shepardson became the guiding light and founding father of DMORT.

Today, DMORT stands ready to respond to U.S. federally declared disasters where identification and mortuary services will be necessary. With the MOU in accord with the National Transportation Safety Board, any mass fatality incident that they investigate will trigger the deployment of DMORT. The scientific identification of the victims, with their prompt return to the next of kin within a structured and properly managed, equipped and experienced environment is now in place for use in disasters of all types with mass fatalities. Co-operation between the US DMORT function and the INTERPOL DVI procedures must be fostered. As the world continues to shrink and air travel in particular continues to grow, multinational disasters with multi cultural and multi political ramifications will become ever more frequent. Meetings such as this where ideas can be exchanged and procedures shared will only serve to enhance the compassionate treatment of the next of kin and the scientific identification of the deceased.

Free topics in forensics

Identification of A. Hitler from cinemato-graphic documents

M. Perrier

INSTITUT UNIVERSITAIRE DE MEDICINE LÉGALE - SWITZERLAND

The objective of this presentation is to contribute to the odontological identification of Adolf Hitler by analysing photographed documents where his teeth can be seen using a computer imaging system. The advantages and the limits of this approach will be discussed.

The disappearance or death of Adolf Hitler in April 1945 remained a long unanswered puzzle until 1968 when the Russian writer Lev Bezymenski published a book entitled 'The Death of Adolf Hitler' which revealed documents from Soviet archives established during the identification procedures. The book included descriptive information of Hitler's alleged corpse with photographs of remaining dental restorations and some of his natural teeth still in the mandible.

What remained of the upper arch was a nine-unit bridge with four abutments on the only four remaining natural teeth, one anterior intermediate pontic and a double cantilevered pontic at each end.

Five untreated natural anterior teeth were present in the mandible and showed advanced periodontitis, as well as signs of erosion and abrasion. On the left, three abutments supported a six-unit bridge while two abutments on the right side supported a four-unit bridge with one distal cantilever.

No x-rays were included with the Russian documents, but a record of the interrogation of Hitler's dentist found among documents in American archives provided a description of his dental history and status with diagrammatic information.

After the assassination attempt on July 20, 1944, five x-rays of Hitler's head were made for diagnostic purpose. These were later located in the US National Archives and permitted several important diagnostic observations as a contribution to an identification.

Examination of these cranial radiographic plates showed that most of the large posterior teeth on the right side were missing and suggested the presence of teeth up to the third molar area on the lower left side. The anterior portion of the maxillary teeth showed extensive radio-opaque material. These findings, among others, were consistent with previous odontological observations. The presence of bone resorption in the lower jaw was also confirmed in the anterior view of the mandible.

Sognnaes beautifully described the identification procedures in various papers in the 1970s and 1980s.

In the preparation of the present paper, almost all of the stills or static photographs of Adolf Hitler examined provided no relevant information as they did not show any 'toothy' features. However a search in the archives of the National Swiss Film Museum (Cinematheque Suisse) did bring to light documents where Hitler was showing his teeth while giving a speech or smiling. These documents covered a period between 1934 and 1944 when, according to statements made by the dentist who treated him during that time, Hitler underwent no further major dental treatment other than that present at the time of his death. The stills were selected from German newsreels, motion pictures on Hitler's life and Leni Riefenstahl's propaganda films 'Triumph of the Will' and 'Olympic Games 1936'.

Standard cinematographic images were digitised through video imagery in order to enhance the quality of the selected documents. Computer software permitted the treatment enhancement and analysis of the documents. The authors used Adobe Photoshop® version 4.0 software program with the following basic hardware equipment: AST, Manhattan S6200, Windows NT, and Agfa Duoscan 1000 x 2000 DPI.

Cinematographic documents constituting a contribution to the odontological identification of Adolf Hitler can now be treated with sophisticated equipment and complex software, a matter both of historical interest and practical value for identification procedures' purposes.

Craniofacial comparison by computer aided device

B. Smeets

Introduction

The reliability of craniofacial superimposition is limited by the subjective assessment of the comparison. In many of the techniques reported, anthropological landmarks and average soft tissue thicknesses provide the metrical basis for determining the identity of an unknown skull.

In other studies distortions in the process of craniofacial superimposition and photographic perspective were studied.

In this research we tried to improve the superimposition technique. First of all we provided a precise computerised steering device, which enables increments as small as 1/100th millimetre on the translational axes and 1/25th degree on the rotational axes. Secondly, we provided a technique to align the videocamera parallel to the skull. And last of all we tried to facilitate the aligning.

Materials and methods

Imaging equipment

One Panasonic NV-DS33EG camera, an Agfa Snapscan 1212 scanner and a computer hardware card used as a special-effects generator (controlled by the Leila 1641F0058 CODEC) were used.

A permanent vertical aluminium rail was fixed to the wall. A mobile dolly was constructed to carry the camera. The dolly could be clamped at any point along the track. On the camera a device was mounted to determine the parallelism of the cameralens to the X- Y- and Z-axis.

Skull handling

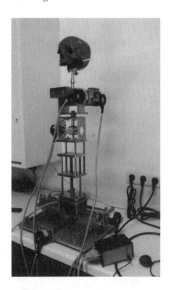

Fig. 1
Skull handling

A specialised device was used to provide accurate, measurable and reproducible movement of the skull in six degrees of freedom. It permits translation in the X, Y and Z planes as well as rotation, inclination and tilt. All of these movements are performed by stepper motors remotely controlled from a computer terminal and incremental data are stored in the computer for future reference. Dr. Brown and Dr. Taylor developed the original device at the Forensic Odontology Unit in Adelaide. Thanks to the VTI in Lokeren we enhanced this device. A computer designed to control the robot was built. A software tool was written to move the skull in all possible directions with increments as small as 1/100th millimetre on the translational axes and 1/25th degree on the rotational axes.

Method

The Frankfort Horizontal Plane provides a reproducible starting position since the initialisation process of the skull positioning robot restores the axes to a standard reference position. Any stored co-ordinates from a previous superimposition can then be used to return the skull to the exact position defined by those co-ordinates and therefore permit a revaluation of the superimposition comparison.

A standard two-dimensional grid was used as source image. First it was scanned into the computer, then attached to the mounting board in front of the camera. The two images were compared for degree of fit.

Tests were also carried out to determine parallelism between the image plane and the lens plane. Therefore a little device was made to determine the parallelism of the lens plane to the X-, Y- and Z-plane. To facilitate the alignment of the photograph to the skull we recommend using a photograph with the face in front view. The problem while aligning is the comparison of a three-dimensional skull to a photograph on which the three dimensions of the face are compressed to only two dimensions. It's very difficult to appreciate the inclination of the head in the photograph. With the face in front view, we use a method based on a triangle constituted by the two ectoconchion points and the subnasal point.

If we draw the triangle on the scan of the original photograph, we can use this still to adjust the position of the skull on the robot. This way the first rough alignment can easily be achieved.

Results and technical discussion

Imaging equipment

Tests were carried out to determine any distortions between the scanner-digitised image of the grid. First it was important to determine the exact parallel position of the lens plane to the X, Y and Z planes. This was done using a frame attached to the camera with levelling instruments indicating the axes. The camera had a resolution of 400 horizontal lines. At this level the grid comparison was carried out and no distortion in any of the 50 tests could be noted. Every time before a superimposition the grids are used to check the camera status. The general layout of the equipment, in a small room with cabling laid across the floor made operator circulation awkward. We therefore mounted cable channels on walls and ceiling so that treading on a cable with a slight shift of a camera position as result was avoided.

Skull Handling

To be able to make the technique easily reproducible we used a remote-controlled, computer-driven system. Incorporated are six degrees of freedom in movement and digital readout of the determined position, which could be stored and reproduced. The stepper motors and gearing system enables increments as small as 1/100th millimetre on the translational axes and 1/25th degree on the rotational axes to be achieved accurately and reproducible. Each stepper motor is attached to the back of a special designed computer. Inside an I/O card with two 8255 Intel chips, which control the input and output functions and one Intel 8253 chip which controls counting and timing functions.

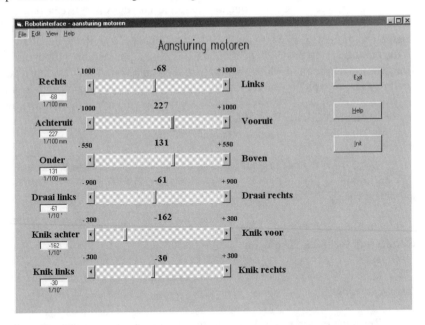

Fig. 2
The software designed to control the functions was written in Visual Basic.

Method

The reproducibility and revaluation of the superimposition comparison, the parallelism of the lens plane to the X-, Y- and Z-plane, and the testing of the equipment to avoid distortions are a mere necessity.

This triangle method is giving us a much faster rough alignment. The fine adjustment necessary to determine yes or no an identity, must in any case be performed by the forensic odontologist.

General discussion and recommendations

Craniofacial video superimposition can be considered reliable provided a number of criteria are carefully observed.

Videographic equipment that provides adequate resolution and detail is employed and care is taken in the alignment of the skull. A sound technique, a thorough understanding of cranial anatomy and soft tissue form and relationships, and total professional impartiality are essential elements in preventing identification of the wrong person.

The overall reliability of the technique can be enhanced by the consideration of several additional factors; some of which merely make the comparisons easier to achieve while others impact directly on the accuracy of the results.

Selection of a good quality ante-mortem photograph will make the comparison of the combined images more reliable. A poor quality photograph can result in an image with poor definition because the ante-mortem photograph is usually enlarged by the video camera. This can make determination of particular features difficult. It is advisable to use more than one photograph showing the face from different viewpoints, if available, so that a series of comparisons can be made before a final decision is reached.

The image of the face in the photograph should be as near to the centre of the photograph as possible. A photograph with the face in the outer extremities of the frame should be avoided, as the proportions of the face will be considerably distorted.

The method of mounting and orientation of the skull should provide accurate and reproducible movement in small increments.

The video camera must be placed in a way that parallelism is achieved. This can be achieved if the video camera is mounted on a stable fixed track rather than on tripods.

Orientation of the skull should reproduce the viewpoint from which the ante mortem photograph was taken.

The optical performance of the video cameras used should be assessed. Cameras that introduce measurable distortions into the images should not be used. If two video cameras are used they should produce images of a similar quality so that valid comparisons can be made.

The ideal craniofacial superimposition involves a comparison made objectively by measurement of corresponding features. Consideration of the guidelines presented above will generate images of optimum reliability that will facilitate this objective assessment.

Further work should address the need to introduce further objectivity into the comparison of the two images using modern shape-analysis algorithms that will further enhance the reliability of the technique and its unchallenged acceptance in courts of law.

The computer-controlled robot, in it's precision, and so the reproducibility of the result achieved, is a conditio sine qua non whereas this method is used to establish an identity.

References

Austin-Smith D. and Maples W.R. (1994) The riliability of skull/photograph superimposition in individual identification. *Journal of Forensic Sciences* **39**: 446-455.

Bastiaan R.G., Dalitz G.D., Woodward C. (1986) Video superimposition of skulls and photographic portraits - A new aid to identification. *Journal of Forensic Sciences* **31**: 1373-1379.

Brocklebank L.M. and Holmgren C.J. (1989) Development of equipment for the standardisation of skull photographs in personal identifications by photographic superimposition. *Journal of Forensic Sciences* **34**: 1214-1221.

Brown K.A. (1983) Developments in craniofacial superimposition for identification. *Journal of Forensic Odonto-Stomatology* **1**: 57-64.

Chai D.S., Lan Y.W., Tao C., Gui R.J., Mu Y.C., Feng J.H., Wang W.D., Zhu J. (1989) A study on the standard for forensic anthropologic identification of skull image superimposition. *Journal of Forensic Sciences* **34**: 1343-1356.

Chee L.F., Cheng C.T. (1989) Skull and photographic superimposition: a new approach using a second party's interpupil distance to extrapolate the magnification factor. *Journal of Forensic Sciences* **34**: 708-713.

Dorion R.B. (1983) Photographic superimposition. *Journal of Forensic Sciences* **28**: 724-734.

Fourmousis I., Bragger U., Burgin W., Tonetti M., Lang N.P. (1994) Digital image processing. I. Evaluation of grey level correction methods in vitro. *Clinical Oral Implants Research* **5**: 37- 7.

Gruner O. and Reinhard R. (1959) Ein photographisches Verfahren zur Schadelidentifizierung. *Deutsche Zeitschrift fur Gerichtliche Medizin* **47**: 247-256.

Helmer R.P. and Gruner O. (1977) Schadelidentifizierung durch Superprojektion nach dem verfahren der elektronischen Bildmischung, modifiziert zum Trickbild-Differenz-Verfahren. *Zeitschrift für Rechtsmedizin* **80**: 189-190.

Helmer R.P. and Gruner O. (1977) Vereinfachte Schadelidentifizierung nach dem superprojektionsverfahren mit hilfe einer video-anlage. *Zeitschrift für Rechtsmedizin* **80**: 183-187.

Helmer R.P., Schimmler J.B., Rieger J. (1989) On the conclusiveness of skull identification via the video superimposition technique. *Canadian Society of Forensic Science Journal* **22**: 177-194.

Ishibashi H. (1986) Identification of a person by the superimposition method. *Japanese Journal Legal Medicine* **40**: 445-454.

Iten P.X. (1987) Identification of skulls by video superimposition. *Journal of Forensic Sciences* **32**: 173-188.

Klonaris N.S. and Furue T. (1980) Photographic superimposition in dental identification: Is a picture worth a thousand words? *Journal of Forensic Sciences* **25**: 859-865.

McKenna J.J. (1985) Studies of the method of matching skulls with photographic portraits using landmarks and measurements of the dentition. *Journal of Forensic Odonto-Stomatology* **3**: 1-6.

McKenna J.J., Jablonski N.G., Fernhead R.W. (1984) A method of matching skulls with photographic portraits using landmarks and measurements of the dentition. *Journal of Forensic Sciences* **29**: 787-797.

Miyasaka S., Yoshino M., Imaizumi K., Seta S. (1995) The computer-aided facial reconstruction system. *Forensic Science International* **74**: 155-165.

Shahrom A.W., Vanezis P., Chapman R.C., Gonzales A. (1996) Techniques in facial identification: computer-aided facial reconstruction using a laser scanner and video superimposition. *International Journal of Legal Medicine* **108**: 194-200.

Yoshino M., Imaizumi K., Miyasaka S., Seta S. (1995) Evaluation of anatomical consistency in craniofacial superimposition images. *Forensic Science International* **74**: 125-134.

Dental age estimation and computers

G. Willems

KATHOLIEKE UNIVERSITEIT LEUVEN – FACULTY OF MEDICINE - BELGIUM
SCHOOL OF DENTISTRY, ORAL PATHOLOGY AND MAXILLOFACIAL SURGERY – DEPT. ORTHODONTICS
CENTRE OF FORENSIC MEDICINE - FORENSIC ODONTOLOGY

Introduction

Age estimation is a sub-discipline of the forensic sciences and should be an important part of every identification process, especially when no information is available related to the deceased. An accurate estimation is of the utmost importance since it narrows down the search within the missing person's files and enables a more efficient approach. Age estimation is of huge importance within forensic medicine, not only for identification purposes of deceased victims, but also in connection with crimes and accidents. In addition, chronological age is important in most societies for school attendance, social benefits, employment and marriage.

Dental maturity has played an important role in estimating the chronological age of individuals. This is due to a reported low variability of dental indicators. Techniques for chronological age estimation in children based on dental maturation may be divided into those using the atlas approach and those using scoring systems. Furthermore, in adults one must distinguish between morphological and radiological techniques.

Dental age estimation in children

Atlas approach

Characteristic for techniques using the atlas approach is the use of radiographs in order to identify the morphologically distinct stages of mineralization that all teeth share. Compared to bone mineralization, tooth mineralization stages are much less affected by variation in nutritional and endocrine status and developing teeth therefore provide a more accurate indication of chronological age.

The Tables of Schour and Massler (1940) have become a classic example of an atlas approach. They described about 20 chronological stadia of dental development starting from 4 months after birth until 21 years of age. Comparing an individual's dental development with these tables results in an estimation of the chronological age.

Moorrees et al. (1963) divided dental maturation of the permanent dentition into 14 different stages ranging from 'Initial cusp formation' until 'Apical closure complete' and designed different tables for males and females. For each tooth an estimation of chronological age can be read from these tables based on the mineralization and stage of development of that specific tooth.

Anderson et al. (1976) eventually determined the chronological age at which tooth mineralization occurred for the 14 stages used by Moorrees et al. (1963) for all teeth including the third molars. The Tables by Anderson et al. (1976) are considered very comprehensive and can be applied for chronological age estimation in juveniles of indefinite age.

Scoring system

Demirjian et al. (1973) actually tried to simplify chronological age estimation base on tooth development. They restricted the number of stages of tooth development to 8 giving them a score of 'A' through 'H' and based the analysis on the first seven teeth of the left lower quadrant. Based on statistical analysis they were able to assign a maturity score for each of these seven teeth to almost each of the 8 developmental stages and differentiated for boys and girls as can be seen in Tables 1-2. Finally adding these 8 maturity scores results in an overall maturity score that leads to an estimation of chronological age according to Table 3-4. All Tables were previously reported by Demirjian et al. (1973).

Table 1: Individual maturity scores for boys for each of the developmental stages as reported by Demirjian et al. (1973).

	A	B	C	D	E	F	G	H
31				0	1.9	4.1	8.2	11.8
32			0	3.2	5.2	7.8	11.7	13.7
33			0	3.5	7.9	10	11	11.9
34		0	3.4	7	11	12.3	12.7	13.5
35	1.7	3.1	5.4	9.7	12	12.8	13.2	14.4
36			0	8	9.6	12.3	17	19.3
37	2.1	3.5	5.9	10.1	12.5	13.2	13.6	15.4

Table 2: Individual maturity scores for girls for each of the developmental stages as reported by Demirjian et al. (1973).

A	B	C	D	E	F	G	H	
31				0	2.4	5.1	9.3	12.9
32			0	3.2	5.6	8.0	12.2	14.2
33			0	3.8	7.3	10.3	11.6	12.4
34		0	3.7	7.5	11.8	13.1	13.4	14.1
35	1.8	3.4	6.5	10.6	12.7	13.5	13.8	14.6
36			0	4.5	6.2	9.0	14.0	16.2
37	2.7	3.9	6.9	11.1	13.5	14.2	14.5	15.6

Table 3: Overall maturity scores for boys as reported by Demirjian et al. (1973).

Age	score	Age	score	Age	score	Age	score	Age	score
3	12.4	5.6	30.3	8.2	75.1	10.8	91.6	13.4	96
3.1	12.9	5.7	31.1	8.3	76.4	10.9	91.8	13.5	96.1
3.2	13.5	5.8	31.8	8.4	77.7	11	92	13.6	96.2
3.3	14	5.9	32.6	8.5	79	11.1	92.2	13.7	96.3
3.4	14.5	6	33.6	8.6	80.2	11.2	92.5	13.8	96.4
3.5	15	6.1	34.7	8.7	81.2	11.3	92.7	13.9	96.5
3.6	15.6	6.2	35.8	8.8	82	11.4	92.9	14	96.6
3.7	16.2	6.3	36.9	8.9	82.8	11.5	93.1	14.1	96.7
3.8	17	6.4	39	9	83.6	11.6	93.3	14.2	96.8
3.9	17.6	6.5	39.2	9.1	84.3	11.7	93.5	14.3	96.9
4	18.2	6.6	40.6	9.2	85	11.8	93.7	14.4	97
4.1	18.9	6.7	42	9.3	85.6	11.9	93.9	14.5	97.1
4.2	19.7	6.8	43.6	9.4	86.2	12	94	14.6	97.2
4.3	20.4	6.9	45	9.5	86.7	12.1	94.2	14.7	97.3
4.4	21	7	46	9.6	87.2	12.2	94.4	14.8	97.4
4.5	21.7	7.1	48.3	9.7	87.7	12.3	94.5	14.9	97.5
4.6	22.4	7.2	50	9.8	88.2	12.4	94.6	15	97.6
4.7	23.1	7.3	52	9.9	88.6	12.5	94.8	15.1	97.7
4.8	23.8	7.4	54.3	10	89	12.6	95	15.2	97.8
4.9	24.6	7.5	56.8	10.1	89.3	12.7	95.1	15.3	97.8
5	25.4	7.6	59.6	10.2	89.7	12.8	95.2	15.4	97.9
5.1	26.2	7.7	62.5	10.3	90	12.9	95.4	15.5	98
5.2	27	7.8	66	10.4	90.3	13	95.6	15.6	98.1
5.3	27.8	7.9	69	10.5	90.6	13.1	95.7	15.7	98.2
5.4	28.6	8	71.6	10.6	91	13.2	95.8	15.8	98.2
5.5	29.5	8.1	73.5	10.7	91.3	13.3	95.9	15.9	98.3
								16	98.4

Based on several literature reports mentioning a consistent overestimation when using Demirjian's technique (Nyström et al., 1986; Mörnstad et al., 1995; Koshy and Tandon, 1998; Nykänen et al., 1998) Willems et al. (2000) repeated Demirijian's study for a Belgian Caucasian population. Statistical analysis of the obtained results lead to the creation of new Tables (Tables 5-6) for boys and girls with maturity scores expressed in years. Adding the maturity scores for the different teeth directly gives the estimate of the individual's chronological age.

Table 4: Overall maturity scores for girls as reported by Demirjian et al. (1973).

Age	Score	Age	Score	Age	Score	Age	Score	Age	Score
3	13.7	5.6	34	8.2	81.2	10.8	94	13.4	97.7
3.1	14.4	5.7	35	8.3	82.2	10.9	94.2	13.5	97.8
3.2	15.1	5.8	36	8.4	83.1	11	94.5	13.6	98
3.3	15.8	5.9	37	8.5	84	11.1	94.7	13.7	98.1
3.4	16.6	6	38	8.6	84.8	11.2	94.9	13.8	98.2
3.5	17.3	6.1	39.1	8.7	85.3	11.3	95.1	13.9	98.3
3.6	18	6.2	40.2	8.8	86.1	11.4	95.3	14	98.3
3.7	18.8	6.3	41.3	8.9	86.7	11.5	95.4	14.1	98.4
3.8	19.5	6.4	42.5	9	87.2	11.6	95.6	14.2	98.5
3.9	20.3	6.5	43.9	9.1	87.8	11.7	95.8	14.3	98.6
4	21	6.6	45.2	9.2	88.3	11.8	96	14.4	98.7
4.1	21.8	6.7	46.7	9.3	88.8	11.9	96.2	14.5	98.8
4.2	22.5	6.8	48	9.4	89.3	12	96.3	14.6	98.9
4.3	23.2	6.9	49.5	9.5	89.8	12.1	96.4	14.7	99
4.4	24	7	51	9.6	90.2	12.2	96.5	14.8	99.1
4.5	24.8	7.1	52.9	9.7	90.7	12.3	96.6	14.9	99.1
4.6	25.6	7.2	55.5	9.8	91.1	12.4	96.7	15	99.2
4.7	26.4	7.3	57.8	9.9	91.4	12.5	96.8	15.1	99.3
4.8	27.2	7.4	61	10	91.8	12.6	96.9	15.2	99.4
4.9	28	7.5	65	10.1	92.1	12.7	97	15.3	99.4
5	28.9	7.6	68	10.2	92.3	12.8	97.1	15.4	99.5
5.1	29.7	7.7	71.8	10.3	92.6	12.9	97.2	15.5	99.6
5.2	30.5	7.8	75	10.4	92.9	13	97.3	15.6	99.6
5.3	31.3	7.9	77	10.5	93.2	13.1	97.4	15.7	99.7
5.4	32.1	8	78.8	10.6	93.5	13.2	97.5	15.8	99.8
5.5	33	8.1	80.2	10.7	93.7	13.3	97.6	15.9	99.9
								16	100

Table 5: Individual maturity scores for boys expressed directly in years for each of the developmental stages (Willems et al., 2000).

	A	B	C	D	E	F	G	H
31	0.00	0.00	1.68	1.49	1.50	1.86	2.07	2.19
32	0.00	0.00	0.55	0.63	0.74	1.08	1.32	1.64
33	0.00	0.00	0.00	0.04	0.31	0.47	1.09	1.90
34	0.15	0.56	0.75	1.11	1.48	2.03	2.43	2.83
35	0.08	0.05	0.12	0.27	0.33	0.45	0.40	1.15
36	0.00	0.00	0.00	0.69	1.14	1.60	1.95	2.15
37	0.18	0.48	0.71	0.80	1.31	2.00	2.48	4.17

Table 6: Individual maturity scores for boys expressed directly in years for each of the developmental stages (Willems et al., 2000).

	A	B	C	D	E	F	G	H
31	0.00	0.00	1.83	2.19	2.34	2.82	3.19	3.14
32	0.00	0.00	0.00	0.29	0.32	0.49	0.79	0.7
33	0.00	0.00	0.6	0.54	0.62	1.08	1.72	2
34	-0.95	-0.15	0.16	0.41	0.6	1.27	1.58	2.19
35	-0.19	0.01	0.27	0.17	0.35	0.35	0.55	1.51
36	0.00	0.00	0.00	0.62	0.9	1.56	1.82	2.21
37	0.14	0.11	0.21	0.32	0.66	1.28	2.09	4.04

Dental age estimation in adults

Apart from the above mentioned techniques that focus primarily on age estimation in children and young adolescents several methods are described in literature that address age estimation in adults. Among these techniques are very fine and relatively accurate methods, some of which are even conservative and do not destruct the tooth substance.

Morphological techniques

One of the first techniques for age estimation on teeth was published by Gustafson in 1950. It is based on the measurement of regressive changes in teeth such as the amount of attrition at the occlusal surface of the tooth, the amount of secondary dentin formation in the crown pulp, the loss of periodontal attachment, the apposition of cement at the root apex, the amount of resorption present at the apex and the transparency of the root. For each of these parameters Gustafson designed different scores on a scale from 0 to 3 and by adding these an overall score was obtained which was linearly related to an estimated age. Gustafson's linear regression formula for age estimation was:

$$Age = 11.43 + 4.56X$$
(Equation 1)

where X equalled the overall score. This technique, which was actually based on a small sample of 40 teeth, has been improved through the years first by Dalitz in 1962 and finally by Johanson in 1971. In 1978 Maples tried to improve Gustafson's estimation method by including a correction factor for tooth position but did not succeed in producing a significantly more accurate technique, despite his multiple regression analysis. Finally Maples and Rice (1979) found that Gustafson erroneously calculated his regression formula and they reported the correct formula (Equation 2)

Age=13.45 + 4.26X   (Equation 2)

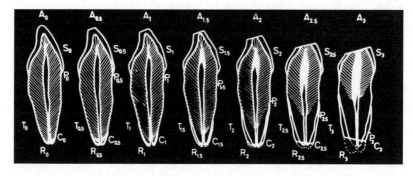

Fig. 1.
Seven different stages with corresponding scores from 0 to 3 relevant for dental age estimation as reported by Johanson (1971).

The improvements of the original technique implemented by Johanson in 1971 are actually the most appreciated among forensic odontologists. He differentiated for seven different stages in stead of four originally and evaluated for the same six criteria, as shown in Fig. 1. In addition, he was able to obtain a multiple regression formula based on these six parameters but was not able to differentiate for tooth position.

Therefore the following formula (Johanson, 1971) may be used for performing an age estimation based on the six criteria, mentioned earlier, attrition (A), secondary dentin formation (S), periodontal attachment loss (P), cement apposition (C), root resorption (R) and apical translucency (T):

Age=11.02+(5.14*A)+(2.3*S)+(4.14*P)+(3.71*C)+(5.57*R)+(8.98*T) (Equation 3)

Earlier in 1970, Bang and Ramm presented a method for age estimation based on the measurement of only one parameter, the length of the apical translucent zone in mm of a given tooth. They differentiated for tooth position, for left and right and for the kind of tooth substrate that was being used, namely intact tooth versus tooth section. Base on a large sample Bang and Ramm were able to present a second-degree polynomial regression formula for the estimation of age based on a single measurement on a single tooth:

$$Age=B_0+(B_1*X)+(B_2*X^2) \hspace{3cm} \text{(Equation 4)}$$

They further differentiated the age estimation based on the total length of the translucent zone. For translucent zones smaller than or equal to 9 mm equation 4 was used. In case of translucent zones larger than 9 mm a first-degree polynomial regression formula was used as in Equation 5:

$$Age=B_0+(B_1*X) \hspace{4cm} \text{(Equation 5)}$$

The regression constant and the regression coefficients for the given equations can be found in Table 7. Care has to be taken to look for the corresponding values according to the total length of the translucent zone and the absence or presence of tooth sectioning.

Finally, but certainly not least of all, in an effort to improve on reported methods or techniques that showed statistical shortcomings or smallness of the materials involved, Solheim reported on his dental age estimation technique in 1993. He measured different parameters related to change over time for over 1000 teeth and selected for each individual tooth those parameters showing the strongest relation to age. For each individual tooth a multiple regression analysis was run with age as the dependant variable. Since both the sex of the deceased body may be unknown and the colour of the tooth may be influenced by changes after death, separate multiple regression analyses were run for each individual tooth including and excluding both parameters. Table 8 shows the multiple regression formulas with age as the dependent variable and the age changes, including colour and sex versus excluding colour and sex, as independent variables to be measured. Among the age changes that were evaluated were:
- AJ (attrition measured according to Johanson's technique (1971)),
- ARA (area of attrition on occlusal tooth surface measured in square mm),
- C1 (sum of cementum thickness on vestibular + lingual surfaces measured at 1/3 of root length from apex),
- CAP (crown pulp area measured in square mm),
- CEST (colour estimation of root dentin),
- EX3 (tooth extracted for caries or related conditions Yes: score 0 - No: score 1)
- LC1 (LOG10(C1)),
- LPMEAN (log10 PMEAN where PMEAN is the mean periodontal attachment loss in mm of a tooth),
- SC (pulp diameter/root diameter at cervical area),

- SEX (gender score male: score 0 - female: score 1)
- SJ (secondary dentin measured according to Johanson's technique (1971)),
- SRS (surface roughness score)
- ST (sum of pulp diameters/sum of root diameters),
- TD (translucency of root apex scored according to Dalitz),
- TID (length in mm of translucent zone in dry intact tooth),

The way in which these age changes are evaluated is described in the articles referred to for each of the measurements and in the work by Solheim (1993).

Table 7: Regression constant and the regression coefficients as reported by Bang and Ramm (1970). Differentiation was made on the level of substrate (intact or sectioned teeth) and length of the translucent zone (<9 mm and >9 mm). (m = mesial; d = distal; p = palatal; r = root).

Tooth	<9mm Intact Roots			<9mm Tooth Sections			>9mm Intact Roots		>9mm Tooth Sections	
	B0	B1	B2	B0	B1	B2	B0	B1	B0	B1
11	20.30	5.74	0.000	21.02	6.03	-0.060	20.34	5.74	22.36	5.39
21	24.30	6.22	-0.119	26.84	6.00	-0.155	26.78	4.96	30.18	4.30
12	18.80	7.10	-0.164	23.09	7.04	-0.197	22.06	5.36	25.55	5.23
22	20.90	6.85	-0.223	24.62	5.18	-0.077	25.57	4.38	25.90	4.39
13	26.20	4.64	-0.044	21.52	6.49	-0.171	28.13	4.01	28.01	4.23
23	25.27	4.58	-0.073	24.64	5.22	-0.143	27.59	3.65	29.41	3.32
14/24	23.91	3.02	0.203	29.98	2.73	0.107	18.42	5.40	28.44	3.81
15	23.78	5.06	-0.064	24.76	4.81	0.000	25.33	4.28	24.75	4.81
25	25.95	4.07	-0.067	22.34	7.59	-0.393	26.92	3.37	26.21	4.03
41	9.80	12.61	-0.711	13.63	12.11	-0.683	29.00	4.23	31.78	4.19
31	23.16	9.32	-0.539	26.46	8.79	-0.511	37.56	2.94	37.89	3.08
42	26.57	7.81	-0.383	21.77	10.19	-0.581	38.81	2.81	38.49	3.03
32	18.58	10.25	-0.538	22.22	9.07	-0.444	33.65	3.53	35.19	3.49
43	23.30	8.45	-0.348	24.34	8.38	-0.358	37.80	3.50	40.32	3.05
33	27.45	7.38	-0.289	23.88	8.76	-0.388	41.50	2.84	42.07	2.73
44	24.83	6.85	-0.237	21.54	8.63	-0.395	30.83	4.05	33.10	3.66
34	29.17	5.96	-0.173	26.02	7.00	-0.234	34.97	3.74	32.79	4.11
45	29.42	4.49	-0.065	14.90	9.93	-0.451	30.68	3.76	27.46	4.17
35	18.72	5.79	-0.082	23.87	5.50	-0.098	20.87	4.79	25.60	4.41
16/26mr	30.25	3.23	-0.018	28.22	4.82	-0.101	30.56	3.00	30.03	3.48
36/46mr	27.39	6.25	-0.239	33.42	5.18	-0.302	30.32	3.66	35.27	2.78
16/26dr	34.73	0.67	0.211	20.43	6.09	-0.182	29.49	3.32	26.89	3.55
36/46dr	30.21	5.52	-0.181	29.91	4.97	-0.102	31.46	3.77	30.31	4.22
16/26pr	27.43	3.64	0.039	25.15	4.34	-0.032	26.81	4.07	25.83	3.95

Table 8: Multiple regression formulas with age as the dependent variable. For each tooth type, parameters that were strongly correlated with age were used in the regression formulas. Explanations for the abbreviations used may be found in the overview above (as reported by Solheim, 1993).

#	COLOUR AND SEX INCLUDED
	MAXILLARY
1	AGE = 24.3 + 8.7CEST + 5.2TD - 2.3C AP - 4.3SEX
2	AGE = 38.7 - 126ST + 4.7CEST + 4.2TD + 0.05C1
3	AGE = 10.1 + 2.3TID + 4.4SJ + 6.1CEST
4	AGE = 8.0 + 7.3CEST + 4.1 SJ + 1.4TID
5	AGE = 6.1 + 9.1CEST + 3.3AJ + 7.3 LPMEAN + 1.4TID
	MANDIBULAR
1	AGE = - 21.8 - 55.3SC + 32.8LC1 - 10.3SEX + 2.6TID
2	AGE = - 24.5 + 4.9CEST + 2.1TID - 7.0SEX +20.1LC1 + 2.4AJ
3	AGE = 19.2 + 1.7TID + 5.1CEST + 3.5SJ
4	AGE = - 28.1 + 3.0TID + 0.6ARA + 24.1LC1 - 5.6SEX + 7.3LPMPEAN
5	AGE = 7.5 + 2.7TID + 4.9SJ + 4.9SRS
#	COLOUR AND SEX EXCLUDED
	MAXILLARY
1	AGE = 25.3 + 7.1TID - 3.1CAP + 5.3SRS - 7.5EX3 + 0.02C1
2	AGE = 46.7 - 142ST + 6.5TD + 0.05C1
3	AGE = 12.1 + 2.9TID + 4.9SJ + 3.9SRS
4	AGE = 14.6 + 6.3SJ + 2.5TID
5	AGE = 14.2 + 2.5TID + 4.1AJ + 8.9LPMEAN + 3.0SJ
	MANDIBULAR
1	AGE = -32.1 - 52.5SC + 31.1LC1 + 1.9TID + 4.6SRS
2	AGE = 37.1 + 2.7TID + 5.9SRS - 46.3SC
3	AGE = 27.5 + 2.6TID + 4.4SJ
4	AGE = -26.9 + 3.2TID + 0.5ARA + 22.3LC1 + 7.1LPMEAN
5	AGE = 7.5 + 2.7TID + 4.9SJ + 4.9SRS

At this time special attention should be drawn to the regression formulas for calculating dental age based on a maxillary central incisor and a mandibular central incisor, both when the independent variables sex and colour are excluded. **When comparing these formulas in Table 8 above with the original reported formulas some small but important corrections must be noted.** For the maxillary central incisors the regression constant to be multiplied with C1 should be **0.02** and not 0.2 as originally reported and for the mandibular central incisors the **4.6SRS** should be added and not subtracted as originally reported. These original typing errors are crucial for the calculation process in order to obtain accurate age estimations.

With respect to the procedures used and the number of teeth included in this major study it is fairly save to state that the reported formulas may be recommended for age estimation in deceased bodies for identification purposes. The fact that some calculations are based on unsectioned tooth measurements makes this technique of particular interest in cases were tooth preservation is of the utmost importance.

Radiological techniques

Of additional particular interest are the following techniques since they are fully based on radiographs. Therefore some of these techniques are suitable for age estimations in deceased and in living persons.

Kvaal et al. (1995) found a method that can be used to estimate the chronological age of an adult from measurements of the size of the pulp on periapical radiographs from six types of teeth: maxillary central and lateral incisor and second bicuspid and mandibular lateral incisor, canine and first bicuspid. The age estimation is based on gender (G) and the calculation of several length and width ratio's in order to compensate for magnification and angulation on the radiograph: pulp/root length (P), pulp/tooth length (R), tooth/root length (T), pulp/root width at enamel-cement junction (A), pulp/root width at midpoint between level C and A, pulp/root width at midroot length (C), mean value of all ratio's (M), mean value of width ratio's B and C (W), mean value of length ratios P and R (L). The results of the regression analyses with age as the dependent variable and the two predictors (M and (W-L)) and gender as independent variables are shown in Table 9. Gender was only included as an independent variable in the formula for the age estimation of the lower lateral incisors because of its higher correlation with age for that specific tooth (male: score 1, female: score 0). The coefficient of determination for the regression also appeared to be the strongest when the ratio for all six types of teeth from both jaws was employed. This coefficient decreased when teeth from only one jaw were included and was the weakest when only mandibular canines were measured.

Table 9: Multiple regression formulas for dental age estimation based on radiological measurements as reported by Kvaal et al., 1995.

TEETH	EQUATION	$r2$
11/21 12/22 15/25 32/42 33/43 34/44	AGE = 129.8 - 316.4(M) - 66.8(W-L)	0.76
11/21 12/22 15/25	AGE = 120.0 - 256.6(M) - 45.3(W-L)	0.74
32/42 33/43 34/44	AGE = 135.3 - 356.8(M) - 82.5(W-L)	0.71
11/21	AGE = 110.2 - 201.4(M) - 31.3(W-L)	0.70
12/22	AGE = 103.5 - 216.6(M) - 46.6(W-L)	0.67
15/25	AGE = 125.3 - 288.5(M) - 46.3(W-L)	0.60
32/42	AGE = 106.6 - 251.7(M) - 61.2(W-L) - 6.0(G)	0.57
33/43	AGE = 158.8 - 255.7(M)	0.56
34/44	AGE = 133.0 - 318.3(M) - 65.0(W-L)	0.64

The previous method by Kvaal et al. (1995) is actually a continuation of the following method by Kvaal and Solheim (1994). The former excludes all parameters to be measured on extracted teeth whereas the latter demands the tooth to be extracted.

Kvaal and Solheim (1994) presented a method where radiological and morphological measurements are combined in order to estimate the age of an individual. Depending on the type of tooth present, the following parameters are measured: apical translucency in mm (T), periodontal ligament retraction in mm (P), pulp length measured on radiographs (PL), root length measured on radiographs on mesial surface (RL), pulp width at cement enamel junction on radiographs (PWC), root width at cement enamel junction on radiographs (RWC), pulp width at midroot on radiographs (PWM), root width at midroot on radiographs (RWM), FL (PL/RL), FWC (PWC/RWC), FWM (PWM/RWM).

Table 10 shows the obtained multiple regression formulas for age calculation with the size of the pulp chamber on dental radiographs, the periodontal retraction and apical translucency as independent variables. A separate equation is given excluding apical translucency where applicable.

Table 10: Multiple regression formulas for dental age estimation based on radiological measurements as reported by Kvaal et al., 1995.

TOOTH		EQUATION
11/21		AGE = 71.2 - 133.7FWM - 56.0 FWC
12/22		AGE = 69.3 - 14.5FWM - 63.0FWC
13/23		AGE = 120.2 - 62.5FL
14/24		AGE = 82.0 - 95.9FWC + 2.0T + 1.7P - 50.6FL
	*	AGE = 112.6 - 85.0FWC + 2.4P - 116.3FWM - 64.8FL
15/25		AGE = 30.8 + 2.5P -96.0FWC + 3.7T
	*	AGE = 36.9 + 2.9P - 102.9FWC
31/41		AGE = 40.3 - 122.4FWC + 4.4T
	*	AGE = 68.5 - 124.4FWC
32/42		AGE = 72.1 - 173.6FWC
33/43		AGE = 43.8 - 139.6FWC + 3.8T
	*	AGE = 75.9 - 174.7FWC
34/44		AGE = 75.5 - 185.9FWC - 105.4FWM + 1.4P
35/45		AGE = 54.0 - 107.0FWM - 97.0FWC + 2.4T
	*	AGE = 80.0 - 192.7FWM - 96.6FWC

* excluding apical translucency

Dental age calculating software

The author developed a software program that is made available in order to automate dental age calculations. Fig. 2 shows the general screen of the program that shows the most accurate and often referenced techniques that are reported in literature. Only those programs are included that really demand extensive calculations. Techniques using an atlas approach as discussed earlier were omitted. Fig. 3 shows the general layout of Solheim's technique (1993) with the parameters colour and sex included. Measuring the required parameters and entering their values into the program results in immediate dental age estimations. Automatic calculating processes avoid calculating errors and time becomes available for repeated measurements and use of different techniques at the same time hereby drastically increasing the scientific value of the age estimation itself.

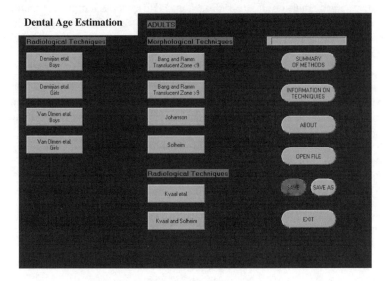

Fig. 2.
Main window from the Dental Age Estimation program showing the techniques incorporated in the program.

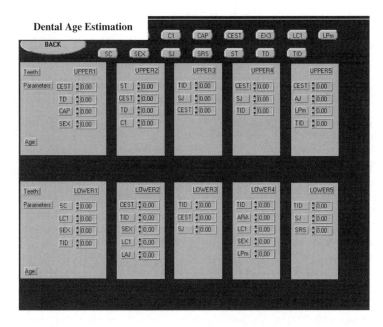

Fig. 3.
Window showing the parameters to be evaluated according to the 'colour and sex included' technique of Solheim (1993). The buttons shown above are help functions.

Conclusion

This review on dental age estimation techniques gives on overview of different methods available, all of which have their specific advantages and disadvantages. The most important aspect in dental age estimation for the forensic odontologist to remember is that he or she should not stick to one age estimation technique in particular but use the different techniques available and perform repetitive measurements and calculations in order to have an impression of reproducibility of the age estimation. Doing so the forensic odontologist will be able to provide an age estimation that is probably more reliable since it was based on a variety of techniques.

Realising that this time consuming procedure takes numerous efforts in measuring the necessary parameters and using the multiple regression formulas for estimating the age, the author presents the Dental Age Calculation program that can easily be used for age estimations. After introducing the measured parameters in the formulas of choice the age calculation is automatically performed. Changing the input values after revaluation of the measured parameters and recalculating the age only takes seconds and allows the forensic odontologist not only to fully concentrate on objective parameter evaluation but also to produce more reliable age estimations in less time than before.

References

Anderson D.L., Thompson G.W., Popovich F. (1976) Age of attainment of mineralization stages of the permanent dentition. *Journal of Forensic Sciences* **21**: 191-200.

Bang G. and Ramm E. (1970) Determination of age in humans from root dentin transparency. *Acta Odontologica Scandinavica* **28**: 3-35.

Dalitz G.D. (1962) Age determination of adult human remains by teeth examination. *Journal of Forensic Science Society* **3**: 11-21.

Demirjian A. and Goldstein H. (1976) New systems for dental maturity based on seven and four teeth. *Annuals of Human Biology* **3**: 411-421.

Demirjian A., Goldstein H., Tanner J.M. (1973) A new system for dental age estimation. *Human Biology* **45**: 211-227.

Gustafson G. (1950) Age determination on teeth. *Journal of the American Dental Association* **41**: 45-54.

Johanson G. (1971) Age determination from teeth. *Odontologisk Revy* **22**: 1-126.

Kataja M., Nyström M., Aine L. (1989) Dental maturity standards in southern Finland. *Proceedings Finnish Dental Society* **85**: 187-197.

Koshy S. and Tandon S. (1998) Dental age assessment: the applicability of Demirjian's method in South Indian children. *Forensic Science International* **94**: 73-85.

Kullman L. (1995) Accuracy of two dental and one skeletal age estimation method in Swedish adolescents. *Forensic Science International* **75**: 225-236.

Kvaal S. and Solheim T. (1994) A non-destructive dental method for age estimation. *Journal of Forensic Odonto-stomatology* **12**: 6-11.

Kvaal S.I., Kolltveit K.M., Thompsen I.O., Solheim T. (1995) Age estimation of adults from dental radiographs. *Forensic Science International* **74**: 175-85.

Maples W.R. and Rice P.M. (1979) Some difficulties in the Gustafson dental age estimation. *Journal of Forensic Sciences* **24**: 168-172.

Maples W.R. (1978) An improved technique using dental histology for estimation of adult age. *Journal of Forensic Sciences* **23**: 764-70.

Moorrees C.F.A., Fanning A., Hunt E.E. (1963) Age variation of formation stages for ten permanent teeth. *Journal of Dental Research* **42**: 1490-1502.

Mörnstad H., Reventlid M., Teivens A. (1995) The validity of four methods for age estimation by teeth in Swedish children. *Swedish Dental Journal* **19**: 121-130.

Nykänen R., Espeland L., Kvaal S.I., Krogstad O. (1938) Validity of the Demirjian method for dental age estimation when applied to Norwegian children. *Acta Odontologica Scandinavica* **56**: 238-244.

Nyström M., Haataja J., Kataja M., Evälahati M., Peck L., Kleemola-Kujala E. (1986) Dental maturity in Finnish children, estimated from the development of seven permanent mandibular teeth. *Acta Odontologica Scandinavica* **44**: 193-198.

Schour I., Massler M. (1940) Studies in tooth development. The growth pattern of human teeth. *Journal of American Dental Association* **27**: 1918-1931.

Solheim T. (1993) A new method for dental age estimation in adults. *Forensic Science International* **59**: 137-147.

Willems G., Van Olmen A., Van Erum R., Spiessens B., Carels C. (2000) Dental age estimation in Belgian children: Demirjian's technique revisited. *Journal of Forensic Sciences (Submitted)*.

Child abuse and the dental profession

J. Kenney

DMORT - USA
FORENSIC ODONTOLOGIST

In the United States, the first articles on the dentist's role in preventing child abuse were published in 1973. In 1979 the American Dental Association passed a resolution encouraging its members to become more aware of their professional and ethical responsibilities in these cases. In 1992 and 1993, additional resolutions were passed by the ADA House of Delegates. They urged dentists to 'become familiar with the perioral signs of child abuse and to report suspected cases' and for the ADA to 'develop resource materials and make training courses available' and to 'monitor state and federal legislative and regulatory activity on child abuse and to make information on this subject available to all members'.

Because of cultural differences and or lack of professional education, the average dental professional in many parts of the developed world has no concept of child abuse. As an example, some of the first presentations to the general dental community in Belgium on the subject of child abuse occurred only in 1994. The P.A.N.D.A. (Prevent Abuse and Neglect through Dental Awareness) program has brought information to a number of European and Asian countries in the past several years.

Simply stated, child abuse is any non-accidental trauma or abuse inflicted on a child by their caretaker (parent, guardian, sibling, babysitter, or other person who is acting in loco parentis) that is beyond acceptable norms of child care in that community. A reasonable suspicion that the abuse has occurred is adequate to trigger a report by the health professional where such provisions exist in the law.

Repeated research has shown minimally 50% of all physical injury child abuse cases present some manifestation in the head or neck region. As the oral cavity and face are the 'persona' of the child, the head and face are often easy targets of the abuse. It should be emphasised that forensic odontologists in particular must be aware of the signs and symptoms of child abuse, as they should be in the forefront of educating the average dentist. The odontologist would also be more likely called upon to complete an examination of a bite mark or oro-facial injuries in a child abuse case.

It can be assumed that the age of abuse victims would be fairly consistent from culture to culture, nation to nation in the Western Hemisphere For all types of abuse the largest group would be in those six and under, or the pre-school child. About 1/3 of the cases occur in the elementary age bracket (1st through fifth grade) and the balance in the junior high and high school age group. Half of all physical abuse occurs in children under two years of age. Under one year, male children seem to be more likely targets. From a year to twelve, it is about evenly split between the sexes. Above the age of twelve, females are the more likely targets due to the prevalence of sexual abuse.

Socio-economic background and education do not discriminate in cases of abuse. Well-educated families hide the secret of abuse, as do those with minimal education. Those who are more affluent however are less likely to be discovered since they have less routine contact with social services and law enforcement agencies. Physicians and hospitals in more affluent areas will either turn a blind eye stating that they 'do not see abuse' or will treat the occurrences 'privately', not making necessary notifications to state welfare agencies.

Risk factors for abuse in children include an appearance that is different physically or emotionally due to birth defect, developmental delay or anomaly. It has been shown that premature infants have three times the likelihood of being abused over their lifetime. Children who generally have poor general hygiene, are clothed inappropriately for the weather, or suffer from medical or educational deprivation all indicate a child at risk.

Those who perpetrate the abuse are primarily related to the victim as a parent, stepparent or sibling. Usually the primary caretaker is most likely to take out their frustrations on the child. They are often lonely, unhappy or depressed due to their personal situation. Stress, either emotional or economic will play a significant role. The abusers were often maltreated themselves as children. Often the day to day problems with living and raising a child or children will wear the parent out to the point of physically lashing out at the child. Parents who are emotionally immature (children having children), or women who are pregnant or in the pre-menstrual portion of their monthly cycle, are more likely to abuse their children. Finally, there is the sub-cultural abuser, those whose ethnic background or religious belief condones corporal punishment or even sexual initiation/abuse as the right of the parent.

Isolation from extended family support will be a contributing factor. With the mobility of today's society, many parents do not have a close relative nearby to advise them as to norms of child development and rearing, or to act as a 'relief valve' to watch the child or children and give the parent a respite. When confronted by a teacher or physician, who inquires as to the child's condition, they will give a history that is inconsistent, contradictory or vague. The history will often be totally out of character with the nature of the injury (broken bones explained by a fall out of bed for example). They will claim an injury is because the child is 'accident-prone' or due to a rare medical condition, but they are unable to remember the details of the affliction or who has diagnosed or treated the child for same. They will refuse to cooperate with a physician or hospital when diagnostic tests are indicated to rule out medical problems as the cause of the illness or injury. Often times these parents will simply walk out of the office or hospital emergency department when confronted by a suspicion of abuse. They will often travel from one hospital or clinic to another that is a considerable distance from their residence in order to preclude detection. In the US and several other western countries where there are reporting laws, a central registry system assists welfare agencies to detect these chronic abusive parents, and protect the children. In general, when presenting with an injured child, the parent(s) will behave inappropriately by showing a lack of concern, lack of knowledge about how the injury took place etc. They will keep the child confined, or insist that only a minor problem be addressed, when there is a visible problem that is much more serious. These parents too will fail to return with the child for necessary follow up visits, and present again only when the child has another injury, or in the case of dental disease, only when the child has acute pain and is visibly swollen.

It is worth noting here that child abuse is part of a domestic triad; child, spouse and elder abuse. Usually it is the non-abusive parent who will bring a child in for treatment of an abuse injury. The presentation may be delayed by hours or days because the non-abusive parent has to find a way to get the child out of the home and to the health care provider's office. The parent accompanying the child may himself or herself be the target of spousal abuse. The old adage, where there is smoke there is fire is exceptionally true in these situations. It is also true that these parents will often present their children with the minor problem in the hope of being 'discovered' by the health care provider so that they can protect themselves from the abusive spouse.

Abuse occurs because there is a potential within the family unit. The parents were themselves raised in a traumatic manner. They witnessed or suffered abuse themselves as a child. We parent the way we were parented, and likewise we treat our spouse or elders the way we saw them treated while we were children. Children who are perceived as 'different' or those who really are such as physically handicapped or developmentally delayed are more likely targets of abuse. A crisis in the family setting often unrelated to the child will often lead to abuse as the most defenceless member of the family becomes targeted. Usually only one child in a family unit will be the target of the abuse, and in some family units, the targeted child will be abused by the siblings as well.

It has been shown through research in the last 35 years that well in excess of half of all physical injury child abuse cases will show a manifestation in the head or neck region. This has also been shown to be true of spousal and elder abuse, although there is little hard research in these two areas and estimates are from anecdotal accounts.

Dentally related injuries include a torn labial frenulum, scarring on the lips, maxillary or mandibular fractures, alveolar/dental fractures and avulsions of the teeth, and multiple root fractures and unusual malocclusions. Perioral or intraoral burns can be caused by a hot eating utensil, food, or chemicals. A petechial palate, caused by pressure from a penis forced into a child's mouth and other intraoral manifestations of sexually transmitted diseases such as gonorrhea on the face, lips mouth or oropharynx ranging from erythema to ulcerative lesions, syphilitic chancres on the lips or gingiva, all can be readily diagnosed by the dentist in his or her clinical practice.

Bruises and welts and patterned injuries can be found in the head and neck region as well as elsewhere on the body. Marks that are red-blue-purple are usually fresh, about a day old. When they begin to turn blue-black they are usually a day to three days of age. Green and blue marks are from three to six days of age, and brown-yellow-green from six to ten days of age. As the injury ages to two weeks, it may take on a tan or yellow appearance. These descriptions are only rough approximations, and depending on the location on the body, severity of the injury and other factors, may vary in presentation.

Finger marks can occur over the face and upper arms. Slap marks are usually multiple parallel marks where often the joints can be seen. Belt marks are usually one to three inches apart, loops or belt buckles or other objects used to strike the child can be detected as well. Any patterned injury must be scientifically documented as one would with a bite mark.

Human bite marks are all too prevalent in child abuse. An adult bite mark on a child must be considered prima-facie evidence of abuse. Bites on infants tend to be in different locations than on school age children, teens or adults. Adult bite marks tend to leave only one arch being clearly defined, while the opposing arch may consist of scratch marks, or a bruised area. They must be photographically documented in a living child. In the case of a deceased child, photographic techniques, use of three dimensional impression material, and resection and preservation of the appropriate tissue all may be utilised to maximise the benefit of the evidence for the court.

Burns to the victim's body caused by hot water, cigarettes, and other hot objects including electric irons and stove grids all need to be documented carefully. Hot water burns to the child's perineal area are often associated with toilet training issues. Lack of sash marks or drip marks should make the investigator suspicious of forcible restraint holding the child's arm or leg under the hot water. Hot water takes little time to produce a full thickness (3rd degree) burn. Only a one-second exposure at 158 degrees F, five seconds at 140 degrees F, 30 seconds at 130 degrees F can produce such injuries. Cigarettes used to burn a child will leave a characteristic punched out or erythematous lesion about 0.5 cm to 1.0 cm in diameter.

A rather bizarre situation is called Munchausen Syndrome by Proxy. In these cases the caretaker intentionally will be brought to the hospital with a parentally fabricated or induced illness. These children may have had a close brush with death such as a falsified SIDS. The parent may have 'rescued' the child at the last moment. Such abusers are usually detected by placing the child in a special treatment room with a concealed video tape monitor. The abusive behaviour of the parent, be it smothering, poisoning or whatever else the parent can conjure up will be recorded on the video.

Neglect of necessary nutrition, clothing, education or health care are all situations where child welfare agencies need to become involved Emotional abuse or neglect, ignoring the child's need for human contact, nurturing, and well being, or verbally abusing a child all can have a devastating effect on the child. Failure to thrive is a medical condition where due to lack of physical contact and bonding with a mother, a baby will cease to eat, and slowly shut down their vital systems. Organic causes must be ruled out, but intense mothering by the nursing staff is usually all that is necessary to bring the child back from the brink of starvation, and a future of generally good health.

Documentation in the living victim is primarily by photography, and should include use of a 35mm camera with a macro lens/ring-point light and close-up capability. In the case of possible fractures, radiographs may be taken to document the injury. In suspected abuse cases the present at a hospital a long bone survey as well as a chest x-ray should be completed to locate any old healed fractures, Time and date of the exam, victim's name and medical record number should appear in the frame of photo itself, as well as on the radiographs taken.

Any time a child presents with a possible diagnosis of child abuse, a full body examination must be undertaken to document any marks or injuries that may be covered by clothing. As odontologists we are of course trained to recognise and examine bite marks. Because of the spatial relationship skills of the average dentist, they too are uniquely qualified to examine the child for signs of patterned injuries and perhaps be allowed to opine as to the origin of a given injury. Full body exams by an odontologist should be at the request of and in the presence of the treating physician. Observing the child's arms, legs, head or neck for signs of abuse is well within the purview of the dentist, if signs have presented themselves on the body.

As dental health professionals, we are not often thought of as having knowledge in the area of domestic violence physical injury. The comfort level of a given child or parent in your practice may be such that they will even disclose abuse to you directly. The acronym P.A.N.D.A. says it all: 'Prevent Abuse and Neglect through Dental Awareness!'

The Torgersen case: After 42 years and 5 forensic odontologists

G. Bang, T. Solheim and H. Strømme Koppang

Abstract

This now 42-years-old Torgersen case has been asked to be reopened on the basis that evidence given in 1958, inclusive the bite-mark analysis, have been criticised by new experts. Only the dental evidence remains today as the police have discarded all evidence. The characteristics of the marks and the teeth will be presented as well as the main findings of the 5 forensic odontologists, inclusive two British, who have reported on the case. All agree that 'it is highly probable that the bite was made by Torgersen'. However another 3 dentists and 2 anatomists have reported on the case and they found that either the bite-mark cannot prove anything or Torgersen can be excluded. The reports have been presented in the news media insinuating that this is a case of obvious miscarriage of justice.

The crime

In 1957 a 16-year-old girl was attempted raped and killed. An old Christmas tree was placed on the corpse and put on fire. Fortunately, the fire brigade was soon alarmed and managed to extinguish the fire before causing severe damage to the deceased. At autopsy, tooth-marks were discovered around her left nipple. These were examined by Dr. Ferdinand Strøm, the father of forensic odontology in Norway. Photos and impressions were taken.

Torgersen

On the night of the murder, a 23-year-old man, Fredrik Fasting Torgersen, was apprehended nearby as he tried to escape the police. As he was just out of jail after a sentence for attempted rape, he was immediately suspected to have committed the present crime.

The evidence was strongly against him as witnesses had seen a person looking like him following the girl and even seen him coming out of the gate on the opposite side of the street where the crime occurred. Faeces on his shoes, pants and a matchbox in his pocket coincided with the food the girl had been eating. Also, in his pants were characteristic spruce tree needles of he same type as on the Christmas tree.

Torgersen would, however, in the first place not allow Dr. Strøm to examine his teeth nor let anyone take impression of them.

Other suspects

The boyfriend of the girl with whom she had been out the same evening had his teeth examined and could be eliminated as the person responsible for the tooth marks. Also an old lag of the police, whose fingerprints were found on a bottle in the same backyard, was also brought in for dental examination and could be excluded.

A now deceased man who lived with his mother in the same apartment building and who has later been accused by the defence lawyer of being the murderer, was however, not examined. Recently, the question has been raised of possibly exhuming that person for odontological comparison with the bite-mark.

Two experts' opinion in 1958

The case was scheduled to the court without any examination of the suspect's teeth. Then he consented to an odontological examination on condition that if Dr. Strøm could not exclude him, a second expert-witness should be appointed to examine the tooth marks and the models of his teeth. However, Dr Strøm's conclusion was that 'it is highly likely that Torgersen has made the bite'.

Another odontologist, Professor Jens Wærhaug, a world famous periodontologist, was then appointed as an expert-witness. Independently and without discussing the case with Dr. Strøm, he came to the same conclusion 'a probability on the border of certainty that the bite was made by Torgersen'. This is a German way of formulating the same conclusion as Dr. Strøm arrived at from his examination.

The dental evidence

The tooth marks were found around the left nipple. The epithelium was almost penetrated, but no external bleeding or subepithelial bleeding was noticed at autopsy. This has been taken as an indication that the bite was made immediately prior to or possibly after the murder was committed, thus connecting the biter with the murder.

The following marks were noted and were interpreted as having been left by the following teeth. The characteristics given below were registered in both the tooth-marks and in the teeth of Torgersen:

-   Mark 1 from a maxillary central incisor with a furrow on the incisal edge. The furrow widens to the distal. The same characteristic was found in Torgersen's tooth 21.
-   Mark 2 from a maxillary central incisor with only a faint furrow in the incisal edge. A part of the disto-incisal edge has not left any impression coinciding with a fracture of the disto-incisal edge of tooth 11 of Torgersen.
-   Mark 3 is a punctuation mark and in some distance from tooth 11. The distance and mark can be explained by the distal higher part of Torgersen's tooth 12 in presumably being opposed to tooth 43 during the bite. This mark has been taken as left by tooth 13 by the defence and as an indication that the perpetrator lacked tooth 12, which Torgersen had. He could consequently be excluded.
-   Mark 4 is a three-edged mark without characteristics and may have been left by Torgersen's right mandibular canine, tooth 43 with an incisal attrition facet.
-   Mark 5 may have been made by tooth 41 as it is found at a distance from 43. A weak furrow widening towards the midline (mark no 6) is found, and this part is more caudal than the distal part of the tooth. These characteristics were found in Torgersen's tooth 41. A faint impression may be visible between mark 4 and 5 but was described neither by Strøm nor Wærhaug in 1958. This has been taken by the

defence as if the perpetrator lacked tooth 42 and as Torgersen did have that tooth he could be excluded.

- Mark 6 may be from tooth 31 and also has an easily visible furrow in the incisal edge. Marks 5 and 6 form an angle, and there is an area between the marks with no impression. All these characteristics were found in Torgersen's teeth 41/31.
- Mark 7 is a possible mark, but difficult to discern. It may have originated from a tooth 32.

All original dental models and models of the bite-mark were secured by the police after the court case. .

The Norwegian system for expert-witnesses

In Norway as in most European countries expert-witnesses are appointed by the court of justice. Thus they are independent of the parties and should act as a guide to the court in questions in which they have a particular knowledge. A neutral approach is mandatory, and if violated may be punished according to the Criminal Act. This is called the inquisitory system or Napoleonic system. The expert-witness is encouraged to stay in the courtroom to follow the court's procedures and even to question witnesses or experts.

This European system is different from the Anglo-American system or the adversary system. Under the latter system, the expert-witness is either the witness of the defence or of the prosecution and if the experts are in strong disagreement, the so-called 'battle of experts' will take place in the courtroom. Under this system the expert-witnesses like other witnesses are not allowed to follow the case in the courtroom.

The court case 1958

The case went before the Norwegian Crown Court in 1958. Seventy-one witnesses and 19 expert-witnesses gave evidence. Torgersen was sentenced, but he never admitted to have committed the crime. The case was appealed to the Norwegian Supreme Court, but the appeal was refused.

The appeal 1973

Just before a possible release in 1973, Torgersen submitted an appeal to have the case re-opened. As the bite-mark appeared to be the most important evidence and as a couple of critical reports had been produced, the court appointed Professor Gisle Bang in Bergen, Norway to re-evaluate the evidence.

Partly based on his evidence, the re-petition was dismissed by the court. Everyone now thought that the Torgersen case would never come up again. Torgersen was released in 1974. The police must have discarded the original dental evidence sometime afterwards, as it is not available today.

The third expert 1974

Professor Gisle Bang re-examined all the original evidence material in 1974. In addition to conventional comparison he also applied scanning electron microscopy and a stereometric plotting technique. The results supported the contention that the bite was made by Torgersen. Also, stereoscopic pictures of the tooth-marks and the teeth convincingly showed the similarities in the mark and teeth (Bang 1976). In accordance with Norwegian tradition his conclusion was 'it is highly likely that the bite-marks are made by Torgersen'. That was exactly the same conclusion as drawn by Dr. Strøm in 1958

The appeal 1998

After a report by Torgersen's private dentist concluding that Torgersen could not have committed the bite, an appeal for re-opening the case was submitted to the Crown Court in 1998. Now all original material was discarded, and 'modern' experts have written critical remarks to the original expert reports. Fortunately, copies of the dental models and models of the breast with the bite were kept in the private files of Drs. Bang and Strøm. These as well as a number of original photos and also the fixed breast could be studied by new experts.

Two British experts 1999

It was now decided by the court to seek advice by foreign experts and one of Europe leading experts on bite marks professor Gordon MacDonald from Glasgow was approached. He accepted, but as the defence wanted also a second foreign expert to evaluate the evidence, Dr. David Whittaker from Cardiff was asked and also accepted.

They were allowed to study all the material and photos that existed and also secondary material such as the stereometric plottings and the stereoscopic pictures from the lower incisors.

In addition to conventional comparison they also employed computer superimposition which just recently had become available. After an extensive report they were able to reach unison conclusion that 'it is very likely that the marks on the breast were caused by the teeth of Torgersen'.

Dissatisfied defence

As Torgersen continues to claim his innocence and the forensic odontologic evidence is the only left to re-examine, the defence is still not satisfied with the conclusions of the experts. Thus they are searching for possible mistakes in the experts examination and evaluation of the evidence. Also they have people that in writing have accused the experts of mistakes and misjudgements. They also have asked for some of their advisors appointed as expert-witnesses to the court.

The 'false' experts

A school dentist in 1973
This dentist compared the reports of Strøm and Wærhaug which were produced separately and found differences in various expressions and especially in the fact that Wærhaug attributed mark no 3 to tooth 13 and not 12. He later admitted that he had made a mistake here, but a mistake of no importance for the conclusion which was based upon the characteristic details found in the bite. The defence still continues to use this mistake as an indication that when the experts do not know which teeth set which marks, the whole report must be unreliable.

A professor in pedodontics 1973
This professor from Oslo without examining the material concluded that Torgersen could not have made the bite. His bases for such a conclusion is the fine reading of the expert's reports and theoretical considerations. These reports did not convince the court in 1974, but is still used by the defence.

Torgersen's private dentist 1998
This dentist also made a report based on the expert reports 1958 and 1974 and concluded that Torgersen could not possibly have made the bite. His arguments were that marks from 12 and 42 was not found in the bite, thus the perpetrator should be without these teeth. Torgersen had 12 and 42. In addition, he noted that the perpetrator should have had a distance between his lower central incisors while he could show pictures of Torgersen where he had no such distance. On the contrary he had crowding of the teeth in that area. His report came before that of the British experts and made the foundation for the defence to invalidate the dental evidence. It also provided the bases for a media crusade to show that Torgersen probably was innocent or at least that the evidence against Torgersen was not strong enough and that this probably was another miscarriage of justice.

A stereoscopic expert 1999

The professor in anatomy, which in 1974 made the stereoscopic pictures for professor Bang, claimed and also later expressed in writing his firm belief that the marks were made by Torgersen based on the concordant details that could be found. Today, however, he points at a number of details that do not fit. He furthermore expresses that according to his opinion 50% of the people in Norway have such teeth that they could have made the bite.

Another professor in anatomy (anthropology) 1999

Also another 'expert' has been produced by the defence. He claims that as an expert on human skin he has a background for understanding the bite better than forensic odontologists. Nevertheless he could not orientate the bite as for which marks come from the upper and from the lower jaw. He also claims that an angle between tooth 21 and 22 cannot be seen in the bite. Furthermore, he still believes that the right part of the lower jaw has set the marks. Based on these findings he excludes Torgersen from having made the bite.

It must be argued that it would be remarkable if the skin by involuntary muscular action and contraction should by accident have given the tooth marks such a shape that they coincide with Torgersens teeth. No one has ever said that tooth 22 shows in the bite. It is also difficult to imagine how the lower right front teeth can bite against the upper left front teeth.

A remarkable case

The Torgersen case is remarkable from many points of view. It is extraordinary that a case is asked to be reopened after 40 years when almost all witnesses and expert-witnesses are dead. It is not remarkable that the police have discarded the evidence material. However, it is a question of how to prove today that he in fact committed the crime in 1957. A Norwegian court will only accept the evidence that can be shown in the courtroom. In other words if you outlive the witnesses and expert-witnesses and manage to have your case re-opened, the state cannot prove your guilt and the road is open to a substantial economic compensation.

The case is also remarkable, as so many experts have been necessary to convince the court; if they ever will. Fortunately all forensic odontological experts have generally been in agreement. For us who have known personally the two old experts in this case, the general distrust in what they did is disappointing and unjustified. They are now sometimes described like they were corrupt and manipulated the evidence to fit their malignant plans. We feel that is to turn the whole thing upside down. In reality, it is the false experts who seem to start with specific views on the case, and do their utmost to find ways to prove their theory. In their evaluation they disregard facts that might indicate that Torgersen was guilty and which the real experts have observed. In fact, we can state that we know the old experts to be extremely honest and correct. They would start all investigations with an open mind. However, when they found evidence in disfavour of one person they would not run away from the responsibility but express exactly their opinion.

The case will set the focus on who may be the expert which the court should base its decision on. What is an expert and what type of formal training and examination would be necessary for the approval? The Norwegian Forensic Medical Commission has taken a stand in that discussion. This is an institution under the Department of Justice that is supposed to read and comment on all forensic medical reports inclusive forensic odontological reports. They have decided to evaluate only reports from persons with formal forensic odontological competence. However, the question who has such a competence, has been decided by the commission itself in the Torgersen case. To further stress the inflammation this case has caused, this Commission has consulted a German forensic odontologist to help evaluating the dental reports. Normally, an unconnected Norwegian forensic odontologist serves as consultant.

The Torgersen case is also remarkable in the way the defence constantly has been using the media to promote a general opinion that a miscarriage of justice occurred. It has not been tradition for Norwegian experts to promote their view through the media. It is however difficult to be quiet when the reputation of esteemed colleagues is questioned because objective incorrect information and interpretations are served as the truth. It remains to see if the 'campaign' will provoke such a public opinion that the court feels pressed to reopen the case.

References

Bang G. (1976) Analysis of tooth marks in a homocide case. Observation by means of visual description, stereo-photography, scanning electron microscopy and stereometric graphic plotting. *Acta Odontologica Scandinavica* **34**: 1-11.

Abstracts of poster presentations

1 Forensic photography in victim identification

J. Stragier*, E. De Valck, J. De Winne

The general procedure of identification of an unknown body contains different stages. As a rule one might say, that ante mortem and post mortem information is collected and used for comparison in a later stage of the investigation. The ante mortem elements are being traced at the victim's family, general practitioner, dentist, health insurance provider, friends and relatives. These elements that will be used as reference material for later comparison, will all be registered on the Interpol AM forms. Photos of the missing person will also be collected, and duplicated as fast as possible to be returned to the family in due time. All post mortem elements are registered on the Interpol PM forms. At the same time all particular visual traits will be photographed. This early photography is extremely important as decomposition of the body may take an early start, changing visual recognisable aspects into non-usable elements. Photography is in that sense an essential part of the identification process.

While carrying out the investigation a number of different aspects will have to be considered: the size of the investigation, the environment, the visual situation of the victims, the cause of death, with a distinction between criminal and non-criminal deaths.

It is obvious that investigations concerning criminal deaths will have a complete different approach then non-criminal cases. In the first case the emphasis will also be on marks on- or in the victim's neighbourhood made by the perpetrators.

To carry out successfully such an investigation the photographer must not only have a sound theoretical and practical basic photography knowledge but must also be trained in forensic applications. It is very important to be aware that most of these investigations involve a multidisciplinary teamwork.

Solid agreements between the different parties involved are absolutely necessary. The involved forensic specialists have to give the photographer clear instructions on the kind of photos they want to be taken. This way they can provide the legal authorities with visual evidence of their speciality.

The role of the forensic photographer, the procedures and sequence of forensic photography and how these can influence the identification process will be shown and discussed.

* DISASTER VICTIM IDENTIFICATION TEAM - BELGIUM

2   Human identification from analyses of the frontal sinus

R.N. Oliveira*; D. Ramos; E.M. Gomes; R.G.A. Mallet

In Brazil the Law that regulates the professional exercise of dentistry backs the forensic dentis to act in the head and neck area, in spite of the fact that we always try to work with a team that involves several professionals.

During the year of 1998 the city of São Paulo was tormented by a serial killer that approached youngsters, seducing them and always taking them to the park where he violated them and later killed them. For this reason he was well-known as 'maniac of the park'. Of two of the eleven victims x-rays were present of their frontal sinus that were taken earlier in time. On these x-rays, measurements were performed and compared with measurements from x-rays taken on the found craniums, trying to establish a correlation between them.

The analysis of the frontal sinus aided in establishing the victim's identity.

* Universidade de São Paulo - Faculdade de Odontologia / Departamento de Odontologia Social, Brasil

3   Cephalometric study

R.F.H. Melani*, R.N. Oliveira, E. Daruge

The present work comprised a cephalometric study of the angles Rivet, Cloquet, Jaquard and Welcker, in 243 individuals pertaining to the three groups: Leucoderma, Xantoderma and Melanoderma.

In a profile study involving Brazilian population it has been noted the pertinency level of the angular measurements for each type of colour skin. Upon these results two main procedures have been developed that are statistically more reliable than those proposed by the other authors.

* PLANALTO PAULISTA, SÃO PAULO, BRAZIL

4   Alterations in teeth of a victim of carbonisation

R.F.H. Melani*, R.N. Oliveira, R. Juhás

We propose to study the reactions and alterations of tissues, as well as of silver amalgam fillings when exposed to temperatures of 200°C, 400°C and 600°C, by use of scanning electron microscope, and comparison of the data with those obtained from the analysis of phenomena occurred in teeth of a victim of carbonisation. Materials and Methods: 28 dental structures (bodies of proof) were studied, which were submitted to the following temperatures: 200°C, 400°C and 600°C, plus 12 structures yielded by identification works in a victim of carbonisation. All teeth and fillings were then observed through scanning electron microscopy at magnifications varying between 20 and 2.000 times

* PLANALTO PAULISTA, SÃO PAULO, BRAZIL

5   Berlin experience with forensic-odontologic age estimation in living individuals

A. Olze*, A. Schmeling, W. Reisinger, G. Geserick

The Institute of Forensic Medicine of Charité Medical School in Berlin has performed forensic age estimations in living individuals since 1992 with a rapid increase in the number of expert reports since 1996.

The legal basis for age estimations according to criminal law is the clarification of the age of criminal responsibility or the question of applicability of adult penal law in cases where an accused's date of birth is doubtful. Civil law cases requiring age estimation involve proceedings pertaining to the various types of guardianship and family law cases. The legally relevant age limits in Germany are the 14th, the 18th, and the 21st year of life. The most frequent countries of origin of the individuals examined were Vietnam, Romania, Lebanon, Bangladesh, and Turkey.

Age estimation crucially depends on the dental status and the assessment of an orthopantogram (OPG). The main criteria for determining dental age are the eruption and mineralization stages of the permanent teeth - especially of the 2nd and 3rd molars in the age group under discussion.

Because civil law does not permit X-ray examinations, an OPG cannot be obtained in civil law for age estimation.

A total of 202 age estimations were performed until Dec. 31, 1999, among them 143 in criminal law cases. Twenty of the subjects were female.

The above-mentioned criteria allow a fairly precise age determination in individuals up to 20 years, while completion of the 21st year of age could be demonstrated conclusively in only a few cases.

In addition to the examination by a dentist, age evaluation in Berlin further includes a clinical inspection by a forensic pathologist, and - where authorised by a judge - an X-ray examination of the hand by a radiologist. These three parts are the basis for the overall age estimation by the forensic pathologist.

We will report on our ongoing research as well as the initial results of the verification of the Berlin age estimation results.

* INSTITUTE OF FORENSIC MEDICINE, CHARITÉ MEDICAL SCHOOL, BERLIN, GERMANY

6 The Significance of dental identification in mass disasters - a case report

P.J. van Niekerk* and H. Bernitz

On September 24th, 1999 a bus load of British tourists, on its way back from the Kruger National Park in South Africa, left the road and overturned, killing 27 of the passengers. The only non-British occupants were the surviving driver and the tour guide who was visually identified.

All the bodies were transported to the state mortuary in Pretoria.

Cost and logistical complications excluded visual identification. Twenty-three of the twenty-seven passengers were identified by dental means, 2 by unique medical history and one by dental exclusion.

The poster will illustrate uniqueness of the identification procedures followed and the quality of the dental records.

* DEPARTMENT OF ORAL PATHOLOGY AND ORAL BIOLOGY, FACULTY OF DENTISTRY, UNIVERSITY OF PRETORIA, SOUTH AFRICA.

7 Bite and sledge marks found in cheese at the scene of a murder case aid in conviction of suspect in high court: a case report

H. Bernitz* and P.J. van Niekerk

On October 10th, 1995 an elderly couple was attacked and robbed at their home in Vereeniging, South Africa. The wife was badly beaten and raped, and died at the scene of the crime. A piece of cheese with very distinctive bite and sledge marks was found near the corpse. The cheese was initially stored in a crime kit container and kept refrigerated by the police. It was only after six months that a silicone impression was made from the cheese.

In May of 1998, five suspects were arrested. On comparing the models taken from the suspects and the cheese bite impression it was clear that suspect 4 had produced the bite marks in the cheese.

After a lengthy Supreme Court case in which three forensic odontologists gave more than 50 hours of expert witness, the suspect was found guilty of murder and sentenced to life imprisonment. The cheese was regarded as substantive evidence.

The 16 concordant features found will be illustrated and discussed. The technique of analysing pattern association and the three dimensional association of the features will be illustrated.

In conclusion the need for further research into aspects of cheese bite mark analysis will be highlighted.

* Department of Oral Pathology and Oral Biology, Faculty of Dentistry, University of Pretoria, South Africa.

8 Age estimation based on the morphometric analysis of dental root pulp using Ortho Cubic Super High Resolution CT (Ortho-CT)

H. Aboshi*, T. Takahashi, M. Tamura, T. Komuro

Numerous radiographic morphometric studies of age related changes of the dental pulp have been published in the forensic literature. In most previous studies measurements of lengths and widths of the root canal were recorded using radiographs. The aims of this study were to capture cross-sectional digital images of teeth for measurements using the Ortho-CT; and to develop an age estimation method by morphometric analysis of cross-sectional dental root pulp as a non-destructive method.

The X-ray CT is an optimal tool for diagnosis of extensive lesions but not for small legions occurring in the maxillofacial region. Arai has recently developed the compact X-ray CT, Ortho-CT, with an image reproductive field limited to a columnar area of 3.5 cm in diameter and 3 cm in depth. Since each voxel is an orthocubic figure whose sides are 0.133mm precise diagnosis is possible due to the minimal resolution difference in the image even when the direction of the scanning axis is changed. A total of 92 extracted lower first premolars, age range 16-77 years, were mounted on this apparatus and scanned for Ortho-CT images. A series of cross- sectional images at 1mm intervals were obtained and the ratio between the areas of the pulp and root at the level of 3mm above the mid-level of the root was used as the variable for regression analysis. The coefficient of determination (R^2) was 0.72 and the variable used for estimating age by this method showed a significant correlation at $P<0.01$ level. Although the sample size was relatively small, and was collected in uncontrolled conditions, the results of this study provide good support for the use of Ortho-CT images of the teeth in age determination.

* DEPARTMENT OF LEGAL MEDICINE, SCHOOL OF DENTISTRY, NIHON UNIVERSITY, JAPAN

9   Ante mortem - post mortem documentation of dental findings. Anatomic or geometric dental charting **

K Rötzscher.*, S. Benthaus, B. Höhmann, C. Grundmann

There exists a lack in the number of international forensic dental experts, in the unique tooth designation worldwide and the exact dental charting by dentists. But there seems to be also a lack in the post mortem documentation of dental findings. The use of the FDI Two-Digit-System as accepted tooth designation in most (but not all) countries enables the identification of unknown bodies in single DVI-cases. Adequate records will not only protect the dentist in cases of malpractice suits but may also proof invaluable if required as means of identification of a patient. Incomplete ante mortem records make positive identification more difficult.

It is not necessary to use a specific dental chart, though it must be clear, legible and understandable – hieroglyphs may lead to long distance telephone, fax or long time discussions between the dentist and the dental expert.

The Identification Commission in Germany exists since 1972, including dental experts, belonging to the Federal Crime Investigation Bureau (Bundeskriminalamt) in Wiesbaden. In single identification cases in Germany the 'Pol KP 16 D' form, and in DVI cases, including not only German citizens, the Interpol PM pink form are in use, both with a semi-anatomic respectively geometric dental part (without any description of dental roots). In so far it is impossible to compare an exact and correct AM information (Interpol AM yellow form F2) regarding restorations in the root-area of the teeth, i.e. root fillings, hemisections, apical ostitis, rests of roots in edentulous cases and implants in the root and/or jaws area.

The German Association of Forensic Odonto-Stomatology (AKFOS) therefore designed and recommends an AM/PM form including dental roots as important parts of teeth for comparison with the AM description in dental records (Rötzscher et al., 1999).

* BOARD OF GERMAN ASSOCIATION OF FORENSIC ODONTO-STOMATOLOGY (AKFOS)
**RÖTZSCHER K., BENTHAUS S., HÖHMANN B., GRUNDMANN C. (1999) ZUR DOKUMENTATION ZAHNÄRTZLICHER BEFUNDE. KRIMINALISTIK 53: 411-413.

10   Estimation of age from dentition for medico-legal purposes

S.S. Muhammed, F.A. Baker, N.A. Al-Mufti*.

In this study, estimation of age was done for 562 Iraqi individuals who attended the Medico-Legal Institute for that purpose. Their estimated ages were between 6 months and 17 years.

Clinical and radiographical examinations were performed to estimate their ages from their dental records. The period of the work was 6 months commencing from 1st of November 1997 to the 1st of May 1998. The results showed that the age estimation using dental information is significantly helpful and supplementary to skeletal examination.

* DENTAL TECHNOLOGY DEPARTMENT, COLLEGE OF MEDICINE AND HEALTH TECHNOLOGY, IRAQ

11   French methodology of Identification of victims of disasters, based upon recent experiences (Order of the Solar Temple, Tunnel of the Mount Blanc)

C. Laborier*, C. Danjard, J.C. Bonnetain, C. Georget

- The presence of an odontologist is to be hoped where the disaster happened, so that he would well understand what the conditions are and how it is possible not to lose elements of proof, which are often deciding.
- An odontologist has to take part (with the investigating commissioners) in the analysis of the ante mortem documents.
- It is necessary that two odontologists be present at each of the tables of autopsy. They practice the lifting of maxillas and write the first post mortem odontograms.
- Meeting of synthesis each evening at the I.M.L. with all the forensic staff.
- The lifting of maxillas should not be missed. It is thanks to this taking that odontograms are accurate and that post mortem X-Ray photography can be done in the best conditions.
- In the lab: drafting of the last odontograms. Full cleaning of the bone pieces. X-Ray photography tests. Drawing up of complete post mortem files for each corpse.
- At the end of all these operations, the identifiers give their reports separately to the magistrate.

* ASSOCIATION FRANÇAISE D'IDENTIFICATION ODONTOLOGIQUE - FRANCE

12 Forensic dental age estimation: intra- and interobserver effects and reproducibility of most commonly used techniques. A pilot study based on non-destructive evaluations

C. Moulin-Romsée*, G. Willems, T. Solheim.

Dental age estimation in children is well documented in forensic literature. Both the atlas approach (Schour and Massler, 1940; Moorrees et al., 1963; Anderson et al., 1973) and the scoring systems (Demirjian et al., 1973) are well known and widely used techniques. The same is true for dental age estimation in adults. A plethora of techniques (Gustafson, 1950; Dalitz, 1962; Bang and Ramm, 1970; Johanson, 1971; Maples, 1978; Solheim, 1989; Ritz, 1993; Solheim, 1993; Kvaal and Solheim, 1994; Kvaal and Solheim, 1995; Kvaal et al., 1995) exist for this purpose but one of the aspects that is less known to researchers is that also non-destructive evaluations are achievable.

The purpose of the present pilot study is to evaluate intra- and interobserver variability and reproducibility of several of these techniques that allow non-destructive testing.

A total of more than 150 teeth of several disaster victims where gathered and evaluated radiologically and morphologically. Both investigators carried out the required non-destructive measurements at different time intervals and independently from each other. The study set-up was blind and teeth had been numbered by a third investigator.

Statistical analysis is performed using the SAS Statistical Software package in order to screen the results for intra- and interobserver effects and locate statistical differences in age estimation between the techniques used.

SCHOOL OF DENTISTRY, ORAL PATHOLOGY AND MAXILLOFACIAL SURGERY, FACULTY OF MEDICINE, KATHOLIEKE UNIVERSITEIT LEUVEN, BELGIUM.

13   A new method of human sex and age identification

R.M. Yusifly*

Identification is one of the most typical issues in forensic examination. Sex and age of a victim is always of interest to investigators.

To identify a person, it is essential to produce, side by side with other material evidence, hair detected on a scene of accident.

In examining morphological, serological and physical parameters of hair, it would be appropriate, to our thinking, to carry on an additional examination to identify sex and age on the basis of a thermal analysis procedure: differential thermal analysis (DTA) and thermogravimetric analysis (TGA)of the hair shaft.

The use of auxiliary methods of DTA and TGA for the solution of the urgent issues of forensic medicine and criminalistics, namely person identification, will make it possible to enhance an objective approach to human hair examination for the purpose of sex and age determination.

* SCIENTIFIC PROFBLEM LABORATORY FOR HAIR ANALYSIS, AZERBAIJAN MEDICAL UNIVERSITY, AZERBAIJAN.

14   The evaluation of morphological parameters on teeth for age estimation using computer image analysis

F. Pudil and A. Pilin*

The aim of this study is to show the possibilities of assessment of morphological parameters on the tooth used for age estimation like attrition, recession of periodontal ligament, transparancy of root dentin, apposition of secondary dentin and cementum using computer enhanced image analysis. The image analyser is a system where human sight, the stereomicroscope and the micrometer are replaced by a television camera connected to the computer by means of digitsing card.

A set of 50 lower canines extrated from dead bodies between ages 16 to 79 years were processed. The teeth where fixed in neutral formalin solution until processing. Firstly, parameters such as attrition, root transparency and periodontal recession on the extracted teeth were macroscopically evaluated using a micrometer. Then they were grabbed to the computer using LUCIA G image analyser (Laboratory Imaging s.r.o., Praha, Czech Republic) connected to a Matroc Comet digitising card (Matrox, Canada) and Hitachi C20 television camera (Hitachi, Japan) and a Kaiser RB 5000DL illuminating device (Kaiser, Germany) operating under defined lightning conditions (5000 K). In the next phase, we prepared the ground up sections from teeth and they were grabbed to the computer as well. The morphological parameters such as root transparency, apposition of secondary dentin, apposition of cementum and attrition were evaluated from the ground up sections.

The image analysis software LUCIA G 3.52 was used for the assessment of these paramters. The software LUCIA enables accurate and reproducible measurement of such parameters as length, width, size of irregular surface, circularity, colour profile and many others from the digitised image. These software options were utilised for the evaluation of the aforementioned parameters. In addition, we used the colour profile of the incisal edge as a parameter for attrition. The feasibility of measuring the size of irregular surface was used for evaluation of root transparency, apposition of secondary cementum and dentin.

THIS STUDY HAS BEEN SUPPORTED BY THE GRANT NO. 4753 FROM THE INTERNAL GRANT AGENCY OF THE MINISTRY OF HEALTH OF THE CZECH REPUBLIC.
* INSTITUTE OF CHEMICAL TECHNOLOGY AND INSTITUTE OF FORENSIC MEDICINE AND TOXICOLOGY OF 1ST MEDICAL FACULTY OF CHARLES UNIVERSITY AND UNIVERSITY HOSPITAL IN PRAGUE, PRAGUE, CHZECH REPUBLIC

Drukkerij en Binderij
SCHEERDERS van KERCHOVE
9100 ST.-NIKLAAS